SAFE

Also by Chris Ryan

Non-fiction
The One That Got Away
Chris Ryan's SAS Fitness Book
Chris Ryan's Ultimate Survival Guide
Fight to Win

Fiction
Stand By, Stand By
Zero Option
The Kremlin Device
Tenth Man Down
Hit List
The Watchman
Land of Fire
Greed
The Increment
Blackout
Ultimate Weapon
Strike Back
Firefight
Who Dares Wins
The Kill Zone
Killing for the Company
Osama

In the Danny Black Series
Masters of War
Hunter Killer
Hellfire
Bad Soldier
Warlord
Head Hunters

In the Strikeback Series
Deathlist
Shadow Kill
Global Strike
Red Strike

Chris Ryan Extreme
Hard Target
Night Strike
Most Wanted
Silent Kill

SAFE

Chris Ryan

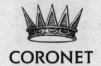

CORONET

First published in Great Britain in 2017 by Coronet
An Imprint of Hodder & Stoughton
An Hachette UK company

This paperback edition published in 2019

1

A CIP catalogue record for this title is available from the British Library

B format ISBN 9781473664364
eBook ISBN 9781473664333

Typeset in Bembo by Hewer Text UK Ltd, Edinburgh
Printed and bound in Great Britain by Clays Ltd, Elcograf S.p.A.

Hodder & Stoughton policy is to use papers that are natural, renewable
and recyclable products and made from wood grown in sustainable
forests. The logging and manufacturing processes are expected to
conform to the environmental regulations of the country of origin.

Hodder & Stoughton Ltd
Carmelite House
50 Victoria Embankment
London EC4Y 0DZ

www.hodder.co.uk

Knowledge dispels fear

Motto of No. 1 Parachute Training School RAF

CONTENTS

1

CHRIS RYAN vs ISIS

The email came through when I was in America.

It was from a detective chief inspector, a Midlands anti-terrorist unit. It was terse and to the point: 'Contact me.'

I did.

I've long since learned not to take anything like this at face value, however. I couldn't be sure this guy was who he said he was. I'd never heard of him before, and there was every chance that he was a crank.

To stay safe, I always make a habit of verifying people's identities. It's a habit I picked up in Northern Ireland. If one of the Regiment guys met a girl in a bar, standard operating procedure was to get her thoroughly vetted before arranging to meet again. Otherwise there was a good chance that they'd turn up at her flat for the shagging of a lifetime, only to find an IRA nutting squad waiting for them. A lot of regular soldiers lost their lives that way.

Clearly this gruff DCI wasn't part of a honey trap, but the take-home message is the same: wolves often wear sheep's clothing.

'I've got a friend in the police,' I said. 'I'm going to contact him now and get him to phone you. If he can confirm that you are who say you are, we'll carry on with this conversation.'

The DCI wasn't offended. But he was insistent. 'Do it quickly,' he said. 'This is important.'

I phoned my friend in Herefordshire police. He contacted the DCI and it all checked out. So I took the conversation to the next stage. What was so important?

The DCI gave me another telephone number. Scotland Yard. 'Call it,' he told me. 'Now.'

The urgency in his voice was a red flag. I didn't know why I was being passed between different police departments, but I had a strong suspicion that the police had become aware of some kind of threat against me. It wouldn't have been the first time. I got straight on the phone to Scotland Yard.

I wasn't prepared for the next question I was asked.

'Where is your daughter? We need her location. We need her number. And we need them now.'

My arse nearly went through the floor.

'Why?' I said.

'You know why,' said the police officer at the other end. 'And you know what they're going to do to her.'

Silence. My stomach turned over. I understood what he was implying: that there had been a threat levelled not against me, but against my daughter, and they were taking it seriously. This was the worst information any father could hear. My instinct – as a father and as a soldier – was to go into full-on protection mode. But I was thousands of miles away. I was helpless.

'Who is it?' I demanded quietly.

They weren't going to give me that kind of intel. The police officer stonewalled me. Maybe he thought that, as a former SAS man, I'd want to track them down and deal with them myself. 'I can't tell you who they are and I can't tell you what the threat is. But I can tell you this: something your daughter posted online has been intercepted.'

My daughter is savvy. I've brought her up to be mindful of her own personal security, and she's well aware of the risks of having a father whose line of work regularly brought him into contact with people who wanted him dead. She had always been wary of posting anything on social media that would link her to me.

But sometimes even the most careful people slip up. She'd posted a picture of me at a book signing in the City. That picture had been seen by a person or persons unknown to me. This faceless enemy had put two and two together and worked out who she was.

I immediately handed over my daughter's number, and supplied her location.

Within hours, two uniformed officers were standing on my daughter's doorstep in the UK. Clearly the threat was deemed serious enough to require an immediate police presence.

Later, Scotland Yard officers turned up at my daughter's house, too. There was only so much information they could give, namely that there was an active threat against her, and that the police were monitoring the people involved. They hinted, but did not say outright, that the people on their watch list were affiliated to Islamic State, and that they were plotting to kill her. They asked her to shut down all her social media sites immediately. That way, whoever was monitoring the terrorists – I don't know if it was the police or GCHQ – could see if my daughter's potential attackers were actively trying to dig up any more information about her or her whereabouts. This would give them an advance warning that the threat level had escalated.

My daughter likes to shoot clay pigeons. She owns a shotgun for this purpose. When the police saw her shotgun out on the side of her house, they told her it had to be locked up in the special cabinet bolted to the wall, which she keeps for that purpose. I'm a strong believer in gun control, but I also believe that a qualified person with a licensed weapon should have the freedom to use it to protect themselves in their own home. You can't sit around with a baseball bat and expect it to be any kind of defence against an automatic weapon or a suicide bomb. But these are not the laws of the land. My daughter did as she was instructed by the police. She was, effectively, almost completely defenceless in her own house.

As for me, I found myself in a position of complete helplessness: petrified for the safety of my daughter, but unable to do anything about this sickening situation.

I told her she should get out of the house, because as any soldier knows, the best way to avoid an attack is not to be there when it happens. I had a friend in rural France. Not off the grid, exactly, but almost. It was the safest place for her that I could think of. I wanted her to get herself there immediately. She would be safe and it would give us all time to think. She refused. A chip off the old block, I guess. 'I'm not leaving the house,' she told me. She wasn't going to let a threat from some scumbag terrorists change the way she lived her life. I wanted to send one of my Rottweilers to live with her, as protection. Nothing doing.

The police went into observation mode. Occasionally we'd get updates telling us everything was fine, but that the threat level was still significant. From time to time I would speak to the police personally. I still wanted information, to find out more about the people involved and exactly what the threat level was. All they would tell me was that they were monitoring the situation.

It was clear, from certain events that occurred over the next few months, that this was a threat they were taking very seriously. My daughter's name was flagged with the police. This meant that, if she contacted them, or her name came up on the system in any way, there would be an *immediate* police response. Over the next few months, she had three occasions to make contact. Twice she had a break-in at her house. Whether these break-ins were connected to the terror threat, nobody knew. But on each occasion, when she called the police, they were on the scene within five minutes.

On the third occasion, she came home to notice a car she didn't recognise parked outside her house. Behind the wheel was a man of Middle Eastern appearance. He was just sitting there, for no apparent reason. She'd never seen him before. Was he putting in surveillance? Was he preparing for an attack? My daughter didn't know, but she was scared. She called the police.

The response was immediate. Within minutes an armed police unit was on the scene. The guy in the car was dragged out of his vehicle, the business ends of several automatic weapons pointing at him. Poor fella. Turned out he'd been delivering pizzas and was having a five-minute break before delivering the next one. But an armed-response unit isn't despatched for no reason. This was enough to tell me that the threat against my daughter was still extremely current.

This terrifying situation continued for a year. A year of not knowing if my daughter was safe. A year of wanting to use all my knowledge and expertise to help and protect her, of wanting to take the fight to these wannabe killers, but being unable to do a damn thing. A year of excruciating worry.

And then, as suddenly as all this had started, Scotland Yard called my daughter to say the threat was gone. She was still flagged, still on the police computer. But whoever had been targeting her was now no longer considered an active threat. The police still wouldn't offer up any more information about who they were or where the threat had come from. Were they worried about giving this information to a former SAS soldier whose daughter had been targeted? Was it for other security reasons? I couldn't tell you. I couldn't even tell you whether the person or persons unknown are still at large, or if they have been properly neutralised as a threat.

But I can tell you this. Of all the situations I've ever been in – escaping half-dead across the Iraqi desert, patrolling the streets of Northern Ireland knowing I was a prime target for the Provos, facing the threat of a rioting mob on the lawless streets of Zaire – none has ever been so gut-wrenchingly terrifying as knowing that my daughter was being targeted by thugs who wanted to do her harm.

Whoever we are, our natural instinct is to protect our family. To keep them safe.

And that's why I wanted to write this book.

We live in a dangerous world. This has always been the case, but there is something unique about the challenges we face today.

I write these words as the UK comes to terms with the

cowardly attack on Westminster Bridge, where a home-grown extremist drove a vehicle into a crowd of innocent civilians, before stabbing a police officer to death outside the Houses of Parliament. Six people dead. Fifty injured. The attacker was a jihadi and in many ways his *modus operandi* was homespun: he used nothing but a vehicle and a knife. No bombs. No firearms. He used everyday, household objects. The kind of weapons anyone with a grudge, or an unhinged mind, can put their hands on.

I've no doubt, however, that the internet, and social media, played its part in his radicalisation. We live in a world where people who want to do us harm can communicate with each other securely and instantly from opposite sides of the world. The security services do what they can to protect us from this threat, but the job is too massive for them to foil every plot. I do not doubt that there are thousands of people out there planning atrocities. But until they have the weapon in their possession, the explosives strapped to their body, or their hands on that steering wheel, there is nothing the security services can do about it. If they make arrests with insufficient evidence, they'll never get a conviction. But they *will* alert the suspect and his or her accomplices to the fact that they're under surveillance.

Bottom line: the bad guys sometimes slip through the net. When they do, the consequences can be devastating.

In the wake of every terror attack, we hear a similar story from the people in authority. 'We won't be cowed. We're not frightened.' Well, of course they're not frightened! Many of them have bodyguards and bulletproof vehicles. The rest of us don't have these advantages. We can't always rely on the authorities to keep us and our families safe. There comes a point where we have to take that responsibility for ourselves.

The threats to our wellbeing do not only come from terrorists, of course. Cyber-targeting, scams, carjacking, house theft and simple, common-or-garden petty crime: whether we want to admit it to ourselves or not, all these are a constant risk in our lives. The 'it won't happen to me' attitude is a comforting blanket, but it's no help when you find yourself in a high-risk situation. I want to use my experience and techniques I learned serving with 22 SAS to help you understand what those situations are, to avoid threats when they come your way and if they can't be avoided, to deal with them effectively.

This book is not intended to scare you. Far from it. It's intended to empower you. To help you take the initiative. To spot the signs. SAS operatives are very good at doing this, and in the next chapter you will learn how, and where, they hone these important skills.

2

FROM PRIMARY JUNGLE TO URBAN JUNGLE

HOW SAS JUNGLE TECHNIQUES CAN BE ADAPTED TO AN URBAN ENVIRONMENT

The information in this book is designed to keep you and your family safe from harm in an urban environment. It is based on the skills I learned and developed in 22 SAS.

But the Regiment's techniques do not derive from the concrete jungle. They derive from the *actual* jungle. It's in the jungle that a large proportion of our selection and training takes place. The skills we learn there are directly transferrable to so many other environments and when we want to sharpen ourselves up, it's to the jungle we return. There, in one of the toughest environments there is, we learn to hone five of the fundamental qualities of an SAS soldier. These qualities are at the core of much of what you will read in this book. They are: personal discipline and attention to detail; situational awareness; positional awareness; blending in; and the importance of training.

Make no mistake. The reason the SAS can work so effectively – and safely – in urban environments is because of the sweat they spill in the jungle. If you can begin to understand why this is, I believe it will make you safer in your daily life too.

PERSONAL DISCIPLINE

It is very difficult for a human being to live in the jungle. You might be surrounded by life, but it's life that has adapted to thrive in that hot, humid, sunless environment. Humans have not adapted like that. We quickly become exhausted, dehydrated and infected. In order to keep going, you need an extraordinarily high level of personal discipline.

That discipline starts with your personal hygiene. You're constantly hot and sticky in the jungle. You need to keep yourself clean and dry in all the right places, otherwise your body can literally start to rot. You have to wash carefully. You have to look after your clothing – your first line of defence against the environment. On jungle training, each guy has two sets of clothes: a wet set and a dry set. You sleep in your dry kit. When the sun comes up, you put your wet kit back on. It's unpleasant and it stinks, but if you don't maintain this disciplined attitude toward your kit, you end up with two sets of wet clothing and no way of drying them out.

This discipline extends to the rest of your daily routine. When the time comes to lie up in the jungle, a patrol will perform a special drill that involves looping back on yourself so you can check nobody is following you. You select a couple of trees to suspend your hammock and poncho, you dry your boots upside down on sticks inserted into the jungle floor and you arrange all your belongings with meticulous detail, so you know where everything is if you have to bug out during the night.

To test their ability to do this, patrols are made to get up, pack up and get moving before first light. It's essential that none of their gear is left behind. In an escape and evasion situation, you can't leave any evidence of your presence. When I was on the Regiment's training wing, I would always return to the previous night's camp after the guys had vacated it. If I found anything – often there would be a stray sock, part of a radio, a magazine off a weapon or just a bit of rubbish – the patrol would be in for a severe bollocking. That level of indiscipline is unacceptable in the SAS.

If that sounds harsh, let me tell you about a time when I was in charge of a jungle training navigation exercise for a patrol of young SAS recruits. We were preparing to do a navigation exercise and, having set out before first light, I returned to the camp after sunrise to do my usual sweep. On this occasion, I didn't find a sock or an old magazine. I found an EMU.

The EMU – it stands for electronic message unit – was an accessory for the radios. It was used to send encrypted messages. It was one of the most crucial bits of kit a patrol could carry. The standard operating procedure in an emergency situation was pretty much that you killed the EMU just before you killed yourself. It had to be destroyed by any means possible before getting into enemy hands. It certainly should not have been lying on the jungle floor, there for anyone to pick it up.

I returned to the patrol and I ripped them a second arsehole. Holding up the EMU, I demanded to know who was responsible. One of the young guys put his hands up. 'It was me,' he said. 'I was carrying it.'

Now, this kid was a great soldier. Best in the patrol. But having the lack of discipline to leave behind that important device was a sacking offence. I looked him up and down. As I did so, I noticed something else. His jungle boots were on the wrong feet. He must have got confused in the dark. It was another unacceptable mistake. I went berserk for a second time. I should have kicked him off the course there and then, failed him outright for these two mistakes. The bar is high for entry into the Regiment, and he'd failed to make the grade.

But he was a good soldier in every other respect. I liked him. I did what I shouldn't have done and gave him the benefit of the doubt. I let him continue with jungle training. He ended up getting badged and joining A Squadron.

When the Bosnian conflict kicked off, he was deployed there. And it was in Bosnia that this kid, who had shown those moments of indiscipline in the jungle, had his head blown off. He was the first SAS soldier to be killed in Bosnia.

I'd been to eighteen Regiment funerals before that. I'd been with some of the guys when they'd died. None of those deaths affected me like this one. I was poleaxed with a horrendous feeling of guilt. I felt that somehow it was my fault. I'm not saying he was killed *because* he dropped his EMU during jungle training, or put his boots on the wrong feet. But I think I knew, deep down, that his personal discipline and attention to detail wasn't what it should have been. If I'd sacked him, like I should have done, he'd have given selection another shot and would have learned from his mistakes. And maybe he'd still be alive today.

Personal discipline keeps an SAS soldier safe, even more so than weapons and fighting skills, no matter where they are operating. It also forms a major part of the information in this book. If you can have the discipline to behave in ways that you know, deep down, are less likely to put you in a dangerous situation, your chances of staying safe are massively increased. An SAS soldier never puts himself in harm's way if he can avoid it. He exercises discipline and attention to detail at all times. He learns these skills in the jungle, but he uses them in every part of his professional life. The habits he learns stick with him for ever. I want to encourage you to adopt the same mindset.

SITUATIONAL AWARENESS

The jungle has other things to teach us. When you're in the thick of all that vegetation, it can seem that everything wants to bite you, to eat you, to suck the life out of you. It can be scary and a lot of the lads become highly claustrophobic. They feel as if the walls are closing in on them. It's hardly surprising. If you're not used to the environment, everywhere you look there's a thick curtain of green that seems to be hiding all manner of unknown threats.

You have to teach yourself to see through that vegetation. To layer it. Part of our jungle training includes target practice along a winding jungle lane. The targets can be hidden among the vegetation. To make a success of the operation, you must learn to look *through* the jungle, dividing your line of sight into the foreground, the middle distance and the far distance. With every step, you're scanning through this thick, unfriendly foliage, looking for objects that wouldn't ordinarily be there. With every step, you're forcing your brain into a heightened level of awareness so that, as a matter of reflex, it picks out anything unusual or distinctive, so that you can locate and engage a hidden target.

Even when you're not looking for targets, you can't let your attention wander. Well-camouflaged snakes. Bushes with huge thorns. Wherever you are in the jungle, danger can be close but unseen. You need to know how to spot it. You're constantly on the look-out for scuff marks on the trail. Overturned leaves. Broken deadfall on the path. They are all signs that something – or someone – has been on the trail before you. Miss them, and you risk walking blindly into danger.

If you think that these sound like very jungle-specific skills, you're wrong. The jungle is simply the hardest place to practise them. When an SAS man scans a crowd for a hidden threat, he is using precisely these jungle techniques. To this day, they are hard-wired in me, as they are in anyone who has undergone SAS jungle training. If a Regiment guy is walking down Oxford Street, trust me: he's simultaneously aware of the space immediately around him, the bloke two metres ahead of him and the guy approaching from ten metres behind. If someone's too close to his back, he knows about it. Almost without thinking, he's constantly checking his reflection in the shop windows and car mirrors. He instantly clocks unusual sights and sounds. If someone is carrying a concealed weapon – it's more common than you think – he sees it. If a person is acting unusually, showing pre-indicator signs of threatening behaviour, he knows about it. His situational awareness is acute and highly tuned.

It all comes from the jungle.

POSITIONAL AWARENESS

Navigation is a core skill for any soldier. But in the jungle, it's a challenge. If you're under a canopy of vegetation, you can't use the sun or the stars. More importantly, everywhere looks the same. If a Regiment guy is navigating the mountains of Brecon, as they have to do during selection, they'll have huge geographical features to help them orientate themselves. You rarely have that in the jungle. You can't even use evidence of your own path to backtrack, because we make a special effort to leave no trace of our presence or passage.

So your navigation comes down to pacing. You're always using a map, and you need to be constantly on top of how far you've travelled and in which direction. To do this, each guy will know how many of his own paces combine to make ten metres. Some will have handheld tally counters – the type you see cabin crews using to count passengers on a plane – stuck to their weapons, so they can keep a tally of how many ten-metre units they've walked. They know that if they're travelling uphill, their paces will be shorter; downhill, longer. That way, when they have to make a decision based on their position on a map, they have a detailed idea of how far they've come. It becomes second nature. You start to have an almost unconscious, supremely accurate idea of your position, and this skill doesn't desert you when you leave the jungle.

Now, I'm not suggesting that you should count your paces everywhere you go. But this heightened level of positional awareness is an important weapon in your safety arsenal. It doesn't matter if he's in the jungle, the desert, the Arctic or in a busy urban environment, an SAS guy's default position is to know where he is and, crucially, how to bug out if he needs to. If you can adopt some of this mindset, you'll find yourself in a much stronger position with respect to your own safety and that of your family. After all, you can't escape a lone gunman, a gang or an angry mob if you don't know which way to run ...

BLENDING IN

During jungle training we wear jungle camouflage. The patterned material breaks up the shape of your body and makes it easier for us to blend in to the background. Later in this book, I'm going to explain to you how and why things are seen – essential knowledge if you want to know how to hide. Blending in is an essential skill for an SAS operative. It's a lot harder for an enemy to kill you if he can't see you. We learn how to harness this knowledge in the jungle, but we apply it in every environment.

For example, SAS operatives are often assigned to body-guarding duties for high-value targets. They often carry on with this work when they leave the Regiment. However, if you look at a celebrity website and see a pop star or actor flanked by a couple of six-foot-six minders in black suits and dark glasses, I can pretty much guarantee that they are not special forces-trained. Any bodyguard worth the name knows how important it is to blend in. If your principal wears a suit, you wear a suit. If they wear jeans and a T-shirt, you wear jeans and a T-shirt. If you don't blend in, you stick out. You become more of a target.

One of your most important strategies in staying safe is going to be blending in. The less people notice you, the more likely they are to ignore you. An SAS soldier knows how to go unnoticed. I want to encourage you to think the same way.

THE IMPORTANCE OF TRAINING

I'm not going to pretend to you that this is something we all always get right. I was once leading a navigation exercise in the jungle, and I got stuck alongside the RSM (Regimental Sergeant Major). It should have been an easy navex, but I made a mistake along a certain ridge line. The further we walked, the more lost we became. The RSM called me all the wankers under the sun, and I had to suffer the humiliation of being obliged to fire three rounds in the air, and listen for base camp's standard reply of two rounds, in order to get an idea of which direction we needed to head toward. It was embarrassing. It shouldn't have happened. But it was also a mistake I was unlikely ever to make again.

That is the last point I want you to take away from this chapter. In the SAS, training is everything. It's far better to make a mistake on the training field than on the battlefield. The same goes for the information in this book. Nobody is suggesting that you're going to encounter a mugger every time you step out of your door. I don't want you to think that every message your daughter receives on social media is from a sexual predator, or that you're going to be attacked every time you walk to your car after nightfall. You're not. But if you can incorporate some of the advice in this book into your daily life, if you can practise your personal discipline, your situational awareness and your positional awareness when the going is good, you will be far better equipped to deal with dangerous situations when the going gets tough. Raising your skills and your general level of awareness by just ten per cent will have a dramatic effect on your safety, and that of your family.

3

STAYING SAFE IN THE STREET

There are hundreds of thousands of reported incidents of street violence every year. These are serious, dangerous incidents. I'm going to tell you briefly the experiences of two young people who were attacked on the street, and give you an idea of the kind of injuries they sustained. These are true stories.

The first is a 21-year-old student. I'm going to call him Alan, but that's not his real name. He was walking home after a night out with a friend in London. They were celebrating their end-of-year exams. His mate had his phone stolen by a group of guys. The two students made the mistake of going after them. The situation turned violent. Alan was hit around the head with a brick. He collapsed, unconscious. When he came round, his mate was panicking and tearful. Alan asked why he felt so wet. His mate had to explain that it was because of the blood pouring from his head. He was surrounded by a pool of it, and had sustained four fractures to the eye socket. To this day, he can't open that eye properly.

Another young man – we'll call him Jason – was mugged while walking into town to meet his friends. Again, he was targeted for his phone. When he refused to hand it over, he was attacked by a group of thugs. He required emergency brain surgery and was put in an induced coma for ten days to avoid sustaining further brain damage from his injuries. As a result of the attack, he had to learn how to walk and talk again, and he suffered long-lasting personality change.

What I want you to take away from this is that street encounters are not just the scuffles we sometimes imagine them to be. They are genuine conflict situations that often result in life-changing trauma to the people involved. They are not to be taken lightly. Alan and Jason made big mistakes in these encounters. I hope that by the time you've read this chapter, you'll know how to avoid doing the same.

THE MINDSET OF A MUGGER

To understand how to avoid street violence, we need to understand the people who do it.

It's possible, if someone confronts you on the street, that they'll back away if you front up to them. You shouldn't rely on this. If somebody is willing to attack you on the street for the value of your phone or the few pounds in your wallet, you need to understand that they do not think in the same way as you or me. They are probably disposed to violence, they are certainly unpredictable and lack empathy. They're not thinking about the consequences of their actions for you or for your family. They are interested only in what they can get from you. If they cause you extreme injury, or even kill you, in the process, chances are they don't care unless it impacts negatively on them.

Most muggers are young. This makes them more dangerous, because their understanding of the world is less mature. They are self-centred and don't have the same ability to consider the consequences of their actions. They may be under the influence of drugs or alcohol, which can increase their desperation and reduce their inhibitions.

But there's something else you need to remember, and it's important. Most street crime is opportunistic. Muggers don't want to work hard. They are looking for easy targets who they know will net them what are probably only small rewards in terms of cash, goods or even drugs. They are looking for low-risk opportunities.

WHERE AND WHEN STREET CRIME HAPPENS

Most street crime happens in the late afternoon and into the hours of darkness.

In recent years, there has been an increase in the number of school kids being targeted by muggers. The reason for this is simple: they are now more likely to be carrying electronic items of value, such as mobile phones. This may account for the afternoon spike in street crime: it coincides with the end of the school day.

The peak in street crime after dark almost certainly happens because poorly lit areas are more difficult to police. But it is also because this is when potential targets are more likely to have consumed alcohol, and so to be less on their guard and aware of their surroundings.

Street crime is more likely to take place in certain locations. These are:

- In the vicinity of businesses that stay open late. We're talking bars, fast-food restaurants, late-night convenience stores, garages.
- In the vicinity of businesses that deal with cash. Betting shops, laundrettes, near ATMs.
- In places that give potential street criminals cover and the opportunity to loiter. Think bus stops and train stations.
- In red-light districts.
- In areas where drug-dealers are operating.

WHAT, AND WHO, MUGGERS ARE LOOKING FOR

For a mugger, cash is king. But it's not the only thing they're looking for. Thieves in general look out for items that satisfy the acronym CRAVED. That is:

- Concealable. If an item can be hidden in a pocket or a bag, it's more susceptible to being stolen.
- Removable. Thieves are on the lookout for items that are easy to take away.
- Available. If an item is in sight and on display, it has a higher risk of being swiped.
- Valuable. The more money a thief can get from selling an object, the more likely it's going to be stolen.
- Enjoyable. Thieves target items that they or other people actively want.
- Disposable. A thief needs to know that they can easily sell something they've stolen.

We put ourselves at a higher risk of street crime if we have items on display that satisfy the CRAVED criteria. In practice, that means cash, wallets, phones, laptops and jewellery.

A mugger doesn't want to get into a fight they're going to lose. They are after easy, low-risk targets. They want victims they can intimidate and overpower. This means that they target people who look lost, lacking in confidence or distracted.

THE COOPER COLOUR CODE

With this information about street-violence offenders at our fingertips, we can start to consider how best to avoid them.

Our first line of defence in this or any other high-risk situation is an exceptional level of situational awareness. When an SAS man walks down the street, whether or not there are immediate threats, I can guarantee you that those skills of situational and positional awareness that he learned and honed in the jungle are being utilised with every pace.

For those who haven't undergone SAS jungle training, I'm going to give you a technique that is sometimes taught to soldiers and security-service personnel to encourage them to maintain a heightened level of awareness. It's called the Cooper Colour Code and it was developed by a former American Marine called Jeff Cooper.

The Cooper Colour Code assigns a colour to our differing states of mental awareness and forces us to be conscious of how much attention we're paying to our surroundings. The four colours are: white, yellow, orange and red.

Condition White

Unaware and unprepared.

This is the mindset that most people will have when they walk down a crowded street. They are oblivious to what's going on around them. They are lost in their own thoughts. Next time you're in the street, check out the people all around you. You'll see them staring at or chatting on their phones, or looking down at the pavement as they walk. They might be eating, and concentrating more on their sandwich than their surroundings. They might be on a park bench reading a newspaper, or talking animatedly to their mate. They might be plugged into their headphones, listening to music rather than to the sounds of the street around them. They will be preoccupied with thoughts other than those of their own safety.

According to the Cooper Colour Code, all these people will be in Condition White. They're not doing anything wrong, of course – they're just acting like most people do. However, they are giving no thought to the possibility that at some point they may need to take defensive action. If you want to stay safe in the street, Condition White is to be avoided. It means you are not alert. You are vulnerable. If somebody wants to target you, they have the element of surprise. And as every soldier knows, if you have the element of surprise, the battle's half-won already.

Condition Yellow

Alert but relaxed.

This is the condition that I try to maintain in my everyday life when I'm in the street. My head's up, my phone's in my pocket.

I try not to be preoccupied. I might still be having a conversation with someone, but I'm aware of everything around me. If there's a gang of youths fifty metres up ahead, I know about it long before I'm close to them. If a car doesn't seem to be driving safely, I clock it. Of course, ninety-nine per cent of what I see is completely ordinary and unsuspicious. I don't want you to think I'm in a state of high paranoia every time I go to the shops. But I am alert.

Condition Yellow is what I want to encourage you to maintain. Relaxed awareness. A person in Condition Yellow, unlike a person in Condition White, knows that the possibility might arise that he or she has to defend themselves. If you're in Condition Yellow, you can avoid potential conflict situations by removing yourself from the threat or the vicinity. If this isn't possible, you can prepare yourself in the event that the situation escalates.

A word of warning: it's impossible to be in Condition Yellow if you're staring at your phone.

Condition Orange

Aware of a potential threat.

This is the condition you enter if, while in Condition Yellow, you notice a potential threat. Someone on the other side of the street is watching you. A man is approaching your car when it's the only one in the car park. Somebody's wearing heavy winter clothing in the middle of summer. There's a shady-looking person loitering on a street corner in an unfamiliar area. You hear the sudden screeching of car brakes, or see a reflection of a group of youths behind you in the side mirror of a parked car.

There may not even be a specific visible or audible threat, just a sudden sense that something isn't right. Don't ignore your instinct. Immediately you enter Condition Orange.

As soon as this happens, you have two priorities. The first is to take evasive action. If you think someone is following you, turn and walk the other way. If you're getting uncomfortable eye contact from somebody, get into a shop or place of safety. If you hear a car screeching in the road, move away from the roadside. The best way to stay safe when there is a potential threat is to remove yourself from it. You'll find more information on what to do in this scenario later in the chapter.

Your second priority is quickly to form a plan. What are you going to do if the situation turns from being a potential threat into being an actual threat? Your plan will depend on the situation. Removing your phone and typing 999, with your finger poised over the dial button, is always a good move. Searching for potential exit routes is crucial. If you think the situation could turn violent, look around for objects you can use to defend yourself or – if the scenario requires it – to make a pre-emptive attack. You need to be thinking to yourself: If they do *that*, I'll do *this*.

It may not happen. With any luck, your Condition Orange is a false alarm. But if it isn't, you're ready to act.

Condition Red

Fight or flight.

You enter Condition Red when you are certain that your safety is at risk. A potential attacker has given you a good indication that he or she intends to do you harm. A gang up ahead is aggressively shouting at or chasing you. Somebody has drawn a weapon, or is trying to get into your car.

I'm hoping that you seldom have to enter Condition Red. Indeed, Conditions Yellow and Orange are specifically designed to prevent this happening. But once you have identified yourself as being in this condition, it's time to act. Call the police. Sprint to your exit route. Action your 'If they do *that*, I'll do *this*' tactical plan. Make a lot of noise. Defend yourself. Strike pre-emptively if you have no other option. Further on in this book, you'll find advice on how to fight effectively in a conflict situation. Now is the time to put that knowledge into action.

UNUSUAL SIGNS AND PRE-INCIDENT INDICATORS

By now, I hope you're beginning to get an idea of the importance of maintaining a heightened level of awareness on the street. With any luck, you'll regularly be in Condition Yellow and seldom in Condition Orange, let alone Red.

To a certain extent, your movement from a lower level of alertness to a higher level of alertness will be triggered instinctively. Sometimes, you just *feel* that something isn't right. However, there are certain indicators that people display, and you should train yourself to become hyper-aware of these. If you notice them, you move to Condition Orange.

I don't want you to think that these indicators mean that a potentially violent situation is a foregone conclusion. It isn't. But if you *do* notice them, you should put yourself on alert.

If you notice two or three of them at the same time, get out of there.

Unexplained presence

Most people are in the street for a reason. They're going to the shops. They're walking to their car. They're heading to the pub for a few pints. Whatever the reason is, you'll notice that it gives them a sense of direction. They'll probably be striding purposefully. They might be holding a package or their car keys. It can be hard to define, but they'll simply give off the aura of someone with a place to go.

If you see someone who does not give off this aura, be wary. If somebody is simply hanging out and doesn't appear to have a particular reason for being where they are, you need to ask yourself what they're doing there. It may be that their presence is entirely innocent. It may equally be that it isn't.

Target staring

If you're aware of somebody staring at you for an unusual amount of time, you should be on high alert. I'm not talking about the occasional glance or eye contact. I'm talking sustained staring. It's particularly suspicious if it's from a distance – from the other side of the street, for example – or if they're staring at you while trying to pretend that they're not. If someone has made the decision to target you, they will lock on with their eyes as they approach. You may also see them checking out the general area to see if there are police, CCTV cameras or anything that could put them at risk when they attack.

Don't underestimate the importance of this. Even the SAS sometimes can't avoid doing it on ops. When Regiment operatives were following IRA bombing suspects in Gibraltar, one of the IRA suspects looked over their shoulder to see one of the SAS men staring at them. They knew instantly they were being followed and the SAS cover was blown. The point is this: when you're targeting someone, you tend to stare at them. If you're being stared at by an unknown person in a crowded area, it's often a sign that they want to do you harm.

Matching your movement

Someone is making you feel uneasy. You cross the street to avoid them. They cross, too. You slow down, they slow down. You speed up, so do they. You leave the pub because you don't like the way someone's staring at you, suddenly you see them again at the bus stop.

This is not normal behaviour. People who are not interested in you never match your movements like that.

Distraction

Generally speaking, people who are simply getting on with their own business don't interact unexpectedly with others. If an unknown person shouts out at you, or makes an unsolicited attempt at conversation, they might be doing it as a distraction. It's the oldest trick in the book. One guy distracts you, the other guy suddenly has an opportunity to steal your wallet or purse, or to do something worse. Behaviour that may be designed to distract you should in fact do the opposite: make you more alert.

Unexplained change in behaviour

You walk on to a deserted train platform. The only other person is a guy sitting on a bench listening to music. As soon as he clocks you, he takes out his earphones and moves closer.

You walk out of a coffee shop with a flat white. The person by the door with an open book and a full cup of coffee suddenly decides to leave at the same time. These are unexplained changes in behaviour. They are one of the main reasons why you should maintain a heightened sense of awareness. You can't notice them if you're not alert to them.

Hidden hands

If someone is approaching you with a weapon, they are unlikely to have it on display. Remember that a weapon can be anything. It *might* be a gun or a knife, but it could just as easily be a lump of rock or a shard of glass. Think of Alan, the student I told you about at the beginning of this chapter, who got hit around the head with a brick. However, most weapons – even improvised ones – *look* like weapons. If it looks like someone is hiding their hands – behind their back, inside their coat – you need to ask yourself why.

Unusual clothing

When a pro carries a concealed weapon, chances are he'll be using a proper body holster or an ops waistcoat. This is not necessarily true of your average street criminal. If they're carrying something they shouldn't be carrying, be it a firearm, a baseball bat or a broken bottle, they're going to need some way of concealing it. Nine times out of ten, this is going to be an oversize coat or jumper. If you see someone wearing hot, heavy clothing when the weather is warm, you should be immediately suspicious.

I would also be suspicious of anyone wearing anything that covers their face. In practice, this means the peak of a baseball cap or a hoodie. Of course, most young people wearing hoodies aren't a threat – many of them are just trying to blend in themselves. But if I see someone who is trying to hide their face, I always ask myself why they would want to.

People winding you up

If you're in a situation where people are shouting the old favourites at you – 'What are you looking at?' 'You got a problem?' – be under no illusion: you're halfway to being in a conflict situation. Don't try some clever response. Understand that you're being targeted and intimidated and act accordingly.

People blocking you

Two guys start walking next to you, one on either side, too close for comfort. Someone approaching from the opposite direction blocks your passage, even if they're doing it with a twinkle in their eye and in an ostensibly non-threatening manner. Somebody's hovering just ahead of you, for no clear reason.

None of these scenarios is OK. If you have the sense that your personal space is being invaded, or your movement is being restricted in any way, or you feel vulnerable on account of where a person has decided to position themselves, you're in a potentially dangerous situation.

People find it hard to believe, but I'm much more on edge during book signings than I ever was during military operations.

On ops, I was always in control. I knew how to blend into my environment. I knew how to avoid drawing attention to myself. I knew how to be the Grey Man.

At a book signing, this is impossible. I'm the centre of attention. My presence has been preannounced. During the event, I'm unable to exercise any of the techniques of situational awareness that have been engrained in me from day one of my military career. My head's down. I'm surrounded by a crowd whose focus is on me. I'm often in a basement, in the centre of a shop away from any exit routes. I'm not in control. If someone wanted to do me harm, my options are limited. If they wanted to come at me with a knife, all they'd have to do is linger in the crowd and attack when my defences are down.

Fortunately, that's never happened, although my training did once stop a crime at a book event. I had given a talk along with some other authors, and was at the subsequent reception with a young lady from my publishers. She had put her handbag down in the corner of the room. We were now both mingling. While I was chatting, however, I noticed that something wasn't right. Or rather, some*one* wasn't right. This guy had come into the room. He didn't fit. It wasn't just that his clothes were different to the suits and smart jackets elsewhere in the room. His general demeanour was all wrong. He wasn't making conversation with anyone else, he was looking shiftily around the room, and he had eyes like a shithouse rat. Nobody else noticed him – perhaps he thought that a room full of genteel publishers would be easy prey – but it was obvious to me, after years of training myself to be watchful, that he was casing the joint.

So when he circled in and went for the young lady's handbag, I was ready for him. His only exit route was through the main door, which was where I grabbed him. He was a pretty pathetic character. I retrieved the handbag and gave him a few slaps. Unfortunately for him, a lot of young guys had rocked up to get some books signed. Once they saw what was happening, they were all over him. He was shown the door pretty swiftly – and a bit worse for the encounter.

DON'T BE A TARGET

Street criminals don't choose their targets at random. I'm a fairly well-built guy. The truth is that I'm less at risk than, say, a petite woman. I'm less of a target.

We can't change our physical stature, of course, but that doesn't mean that our chances of being attacked on the street are fixed. There are things that we can do to cut the risk and make ourselves safer.

Be inconspicuous

This is rule number one. Just as you need to be on the lookout for conspicuous potential threats, so your chances of being at the receiving end of an attack are increased if you stick out from the crowd. In practice, this means:

- Don't dress like a tourist. Tourists are common targets for street violence, because they often carry substantial quantities of cash with them. The plainer you dress, the less noticeable you are.
- Don't wear obviously expensive jewellery or watches.
- Avoid being smartly dressed in an area where most people aren't. If it's not possible, consider wearing a tatty coat to cover your smart clothes.
- Don't keep looking up at tall buildings, or staring at impressive sights. Act like nothing's a big deal, otherwise you're marking yourself out.

Appear confident

Being inconspicuous is not the same as being shy. Far from it. If you're shuffling down the street with your head lowered, or looking anxiously about, it's much more likely that a potential attacker will zone in on you. If you appear vulnerable, they'll sense it. You need to stand tall, with your head raised and your eyes straight ahead. Walk briskly and with purpose. Look sure of yourself. Look alert.

Stick to well-lit, busy areas

This is common sense, but it's amazing how often people ignore it. You are massively more likely to encounter street violence in poorly lit, unpopulated parts of town. Criminals are drawn to these areas because it makes their job a lot easier. The cover of darkness gives them the element of surprise and it stops them being recognised.

Plan your route

If you have to keep stopping, checking your phone or a map, asking directions, looking around for street signs, you're going to look less confident and draw attention to yourself. If you get lost, you're more likely to find yourself in dodgy areas. Even for small journeys in familiar locations, I always make sure I know my route before I set out.

Put your phone away

I'm not saying you should leave it at home – phones are incredibly useful tools when it comes to staying safe – but if you're walking down the street, it should be in your pocket not your hand. If you're using your phone, not only do you have an expensive, easily stealable item on full display, you're broadcasting to any potential attacker that you're not focusing on your surroundings. You're making yourself an obvious, easy target.

I can honestly say I've never sent a text message while walking, for precisely this reason. I wouldn't even walk down the street with headphones in: they compromise my situational awareness and they make it obvious that I'm carrying a device worth stealing. If you must listen to music, use one earbud – that way you're not compromising your senses so much.

Carry your bag properly

If it's a handbag, have the strap across your chest and your hand over the fastening. If it's a rucksack, use both straps not just one. If your bag can be quickly grabbed, you're an obvious target for an opportunistic criminal.

Wear clothes and shoes you can run in

High heels might look good, but they're a beacon for street attackers, because a person in high heels can't easily run away. Put them in your bag and wear a pair of trainers to get from A to B. For the same reason, I'd always recommend that a woman considers wearing trousers instead of long dresses if she's worried about street safety.

Walk with another person

You're much more likely to be attacked if you're walking by yourself. Walking in pairs is safer. Walking in larger groups is even better.

Use alcohol sensibly

If you're staggering down the street, reeling drunk, you're asking for trouble. Street attackers will know that your response times will be low, your coordination will be compromised and your situational awareness will be almost zero. If you've been out on the booze, get a cab home or stick with your mates.

BE WARY OF ROUTINES

In the jungle, if you want to catch an animal for food, your first job is to identify an animal trail. This is the path left by various animals as they move from their den to their food or water source and back. They are creatures of habit. It means you know where they're going to be, and where to strike.

An SAS team will put this knowledge into action on operations. If they're targeting a terror suspect, first they'll put in surveillance. They'll build up a picture of their target's daily routine, so they know when and where is the best time to hit them.

Criminals do this, too. It's why a high proportion of street attacks take place close to the victim's home. They watch you as you leave your house to go to work. They make a note of that moment when you're standing by your car, searching for your keys. Those moments when you are at your most vulnerable.

Our situational awareness tends to be weakest when we're in areas we know well, doing things we're used to doing. In fact, this is when we should be at our most alert. We should break up our routines and avoid this tendency to assume that, just because an incident hasn't yet occurred on our doorstep, it never will. It's hardwired in me always to leave the house at different times and to take different routes to the same locations. I make a point of maintaining a heightened level of awareness when I'm in familiar locations.

USE THE PAVEMENT TACTICALLY

When you're walking down the street, you can reduce your chance of being attacked simply by choosing which part of the pavement to occupy.

Face oncoming traffic

If you walk on the side of the road that faces oncoming traffic, you can avoid kerb crawlers. In the UK, this means walking on the right-hand side of the road.

If you can't do this for any reason, and a vehicle pulls up alongside you making you feel unsafe, run the other way: you can turn to face the opposite direction much more quickly than a car can.

Walk in the centre of the pavement

Avoiding the edge of the pavement means you're less at risk from people lurking in doorways on one side, and from passing cars on the other.

Make wide corner turns

When turning a corner, don't hug the wall. Attackers often position themselves at street corners so they can hit you hard and fast. Putting a few feet between you and them gives you a couple of seconds extra response time that can make a genuine difference. Use the same technique if you're walking round parked cars.

HOW TO CHECK IF YOU'RE BEING FOLLOWED

Being followed is a horrible sensation and a dangerous scenario. People seldom follow others for innocent reasons. It can sometimes be difficult to establish that you *are* being followed. Here are some tips for doing that.

Firstly, don't look over your shoulder. This will alert the person following you and cause them to drop back, so it'll become harder for you to identify them.

Make use of reflective surfaces to see what's going on behind you. In practice, this means the wing mirrors of parked cars and shop windows.

Slow down. Speed up. Slow down again. If the person you're concerned about matches your movement, they're following you.

Stop. Bend down to do up your shoelaces. Look at a shop window display. If they stop too, they're following you.

Take an unusual route. Double back on yourself to end up where you started. If they do the same, it's suspicious.

WHAT TO DO IF YOU'RE BEING FOLLOWED
OR FEEL OTHERWISE THREATENED

If you're being followed, or feel at all threatened on the street – if, that is, you've entered Condition Orange – your priority should always be to remove yourself from the potential conflict situation. Run. There is no shame in this. Any soldier will tell you that the best way to avoid being killed in a fight is to avoid the fight itself, if you possibly can. So if you're in a bar and a big drunk fella is looking for trouble, remove yourself. If you're walking down the street and there's a gang up ahead looking lairy, get out of there.

I always avoid conflict if possible. I was in a small town in France one evening, and a bunch of sixteen-year-olds were approaching from the other direction. I could tell that one of them was up for a bit of aggro. He was maintaining aggressive eye contact with me. I crossed the street. He did the same. He called out to me in French, asking if I had the time. I told him I didn't, shutting down the conversation quickly and concentrating on getting away from the gang. Almost immediately, the kid spat at me.

I evaluated my options. There was only going to be one winner in a fist fight between me and him, and it wasn't going to be the boozed-up sixteen-year-old. But that didn't mean that the smart call was to lay in to him. He could easily have been carrying a knife or another concealed weapon, whereas I was unarmed. More to the point, if I'd attacked this kid pre-emptively, I'd then have had the rest of them to deal with. They'd have been on me like a pack of terriers and that's a fight nobody's going to win, SAS or not.

I turned and ran. Conflict avoided. Personal safety no longer at risk. Sometimes you just have to pick your battles.

On that occasion, I knew that I was entering a conflict situation. Sometimes you're not sure. If running doesn't seem to be an option, here are some tips. You will need to adjust them according to the specifics of the situation.

Dial 999

Or whatever the emergency number is in your region. Do this especially if you're a lone female being followed, and do it ostentatiously so your pursuer can see what you're doing. Keep walking as you speak to the police, and give them your location.

If you're unsure that the threat is going to develop, you can dial the number, but you don't have to press send. Just keep your finger on that button ready to do so if things escalate.

Get to a crowded area

It's common sense that criminals are less likely to attack where they're more likely to be seen. If you can move to an area of high population density – especially an area with CCTV cameras – you reduce your risk of coming to harm. A good strategy is to run into a shop. Don't hesitate to make people understand that you feel under threat. There is safety in numbers.

By contrast, never head toward deserted areas, dark areas, down dead-end streets or into rural areas.

Don't go home

If someone's following you, you mustn't lead them to your house, particularly if you live alone. Instead, head for friends, family or neighbours – you want somewhere you know there will be people to let you in and protect you.

Avoid eye contact

Staring is aggressive. If a potential attacker is on the edge, it can be what forces him or her to confront you. If you do make accidental eye contact, look away slowly, not suddenly. Don't make yourself appear nervous.

Remove your car keys

They make effective incidental weapons, if that's what it comes to. If you have them in your hand and you're heading for your vehicle, it means you can get in and away quickly.

Drop your purse

Or wallet. It may be that it's all the person following you is after. Much better to lose it than compromise your safety.

Look a bit crazy

Or a bit disgusting. This can be a high-risk strategy, because you'll be breaking the cardinal rule of not drawing attention to yourself. But it can be a useful tactic that makes use of basic human psychology: just as you want to avoid sitting next to the nutter on the bus, so a potential attacker might be put off having anything to do with you if you start muttering to yourself, picking your nose or scratching your armpit.

Make a hell of a noise

If you suddenly start screaming and shouting, there's a good chance your pursuer will be scared off. It's a good idea to carry an ordinary whistle: you can use it to grab people's attention and it's much louder – and easier – than shouting.

Avoid inflammatory language

'What are you looking at?' 'What's your problem?' 'Do you really want to do this?' These are not good things to say. They sound threatening and they invite escalation. If you have to engage verbally, use language that calms the situation. 'Come on, fellas, I'm in a rush to get home.' 'I don't want any trouble, guys.' 'I just want to get on my way.'

THE BOTTOM LINE: WHAT TO DO IN A CONFLICT SITUATION IN THE STREET

Later in this book, I'm going to give you some fighting tips, but I want you to understand that conflict and violence should always be a last resort. I don't care if you're big. I don't care if you're good at fighting. I don't even care if you're carrying something that can be used as a weapon. Fights are unpredictable. Often, they don't turn out the way you expect them to.

If a criminal demands your wallet, or your mobile, or your bag, or your watch, or your jewellery, or any material item: give it to him. I can't emphasise this enough. Money and iPhones are replaceable. Lives aren't. Ninety-nine times out of a hundred, if you give a street criminal what they want, they'll take it and get out of there.

At the beginning of this chapter, I told you about Alan and Jason, who both sustained life-changing injuries as a result of a mugging. Now, make no mistake: Alan and Jason were the victims, and the scumbags who attacked them were common criminals. In both instances, however, the victims or their friends either refused to hand over their belongings, or went after the gang who robbed them. I'm sure we all understand their motivation, but it's the wrong call. You should always prioritise your personal safety above your belongings or your desire to retaliate.

There are ways of cutting your losses, however. In the course of my career, I've found myself in many places where I know street crime is an active problem. In these instances, I always carry a dummy wallet containing a few notes. I also sometimes take the precaution of carrying an old phone that I can afford to lose. Most of the time, handing these over will satisfy a mugger. In the meantime, I carry larger quantities of cash or items of value in places where muggers are less inclined to look: inside my shoe or in my underwear.

Sometimes a street criminal doesn't want your wallet. Sometimes they want a fight. If you sense that violence is imminent, you must do everything possible to avoid it. Run if you can. Complete that 999 call. Make a lot of noise. Shouting 'help' is often not a very effective strategy – passers-by can be apathetic to other people's peril, or scared of getting involved. A better move is to shout 'fire'. It gets people's attention and causes a moment of distraction that you might be able to use to your advantage.

Another way of alerting people to your predicament is to set off car alarms. If I find myself in Condition Orange, I'll make myself aware of any expensive-looking parked vehicles. They are likely to have car alarms. If I find myself entering a conflict situation, I wouldn't hesitate to kick the doors of those vehicles very hard to set off the alarms, in order to spook my aggressors and encourage people to come out to investigate. I'd do it to several vehicles if possible, and worry about the damage later.

Only if violence is truly unavoidable should you fight back. If you do so, you need to make sure that your own violence is effective. If it's not, you're in trouble. You'll find some tips on this later in the book.

Much of the advice in this chapter centres on the importance of being aware of people who stick out, and of taking pains not to be conspicuous yourself. Clothing and general appearance is a massive part of that. I learned a lot about this during the years I served in Northern Ireland at the height of the Troubles. The SAS worked undercover on the streets of the Province, and it was crucial to our own safety that members of the Provisional IRA couldn't recognise us.

This was a potential problem. In their down time, most SAS soldiers tended to dress in a similar fashion. Think desert boots, jeans and Lacoste T-shirts, so they could show off their massive, muscular arms! It was pretty much an unofficial uniform, but it came with its set of problems. If you're walking down the street and you see a guy coming the other way looking unusually big and strong, you'll probably notice him. If the SAS guys walked through the streets of Belfast in this unofficial uniform, they'd stick out.

So, when we were on covert ops, we had to disguise ourselves.

14 Intelligence Company – also known as the Det – were a special forces surveillance unit operating in the Province. One of their jobs was to take covert photographs of low-ranking members of the IRA so that we could study their clothes and hairstyles. There was a board at our military base where all these pictures were pinned up, and we examined them very hard. Fashions and hairstyles change over time, and it's easy to get it wrong when you're trying to blend in. During my time in the Province, a lot of the young lads had permed hair, grown long into a mullet. Not exactly how we Regiment boys wanted to wear our hair, but we were prepared to do so if it kept us safe.

There was also a box – we called it the Det box – stuffed full of old, second-hand clothes. The Regiment guys were a pretty well-dressed bunch most of the time, but if we wanted to remain invisible on the streets, we'd take skanky old clothes from the Det box and dress down.

Our weapons and radios, which we took with us pretty much every time we left camp, posed another problem. They were hard to conceal unless you wore very baggy clothes. Some of the guys experimented with bum bags – there was a particular type just the right size for a handgun, with a velcro front that could be ripped down for easy access. But these were not common items in Northern Ireland at the time, so they made the wearer more conspicuous, not less. (To this day, whenever I see someone wearing a bum bag, my eyes are immediately drawn to it and I find myself looking for other signs that the person wearing it is a tourist, and nothing more sinister.) Eventually we tended to settle on a rucksack. Not a flash, expensive North Face one, but a cheap, beaten-up, coarse canvas bag. Big enough to secrete a radio and a weapon, but completely unremarkable in every way.

No matter what pains you took to make sure you blended in, however, your appearance could still put you at risk. I remember one day doing an orientation exercise with a bunch of the guys. We would use these exercises firstly to drive around the Province, getting our bearings, learning the roads and the junctions. Then we would ditch our vehicles and walk round some of the towns and villages, so that we had a sense of the area. On this particular occasion, we'd woken up to a grey, cold day. A mate of mine had taken a T-shirt and a thick jacket from the Det box. He was wearing this as we started pounding the streets of a small town that we knew to be riddled with IRA members and sympathisers. As we were walking, however, the clouds parted and the sun came out. It was very hot. My mate removed his jacket.

Bad idea. On his forearm, he had the regimental tattoo of the Parachute Regiment – a set of black wings with a crown in the centre. Military tattoos were a big thing back then. Guys would pass into their regiment at the age of eighteen, full of testosterone and proud of their achievement, and get inked up, not understanding that this could be a hindrance if they ever had to engage in covert ops. (Down the line, they'd sometimes try to have the tattoos lasered off, but this just left a white mark in the shape of their regimental insignia.)

If anything was likely to mark him out as a British soldier, it was a Para tattoo. Even if it didn't identify him as a member of the SAS, the Paras were almost as hated by the IRA. I got him to put his jacket back on, quickly.

Only now we had another problem. Any IRA member worth their salt would have been doing *exactly* what I'm encouraging you to do: maintaining a heightened level of awareness for anyone or anything that struck them as unusual. My mate was wearing a heavy jacket in hot sunshine. As we walked through that heavily Provo town, we started to feel eyes following us.

And not only eyes. It took only a few minutes for us to clock that we were being trailed by a bunch of guys whose clothes, swagger and general demeanour told us they were IRA lads, wanting to know more about these two strangers in their town, one of them unconventionally dressed. Our only option was to get out of there. Fortunately, our positional awareness was sufficiently good that we could find our way back to our vehicle through relatively well-populated areas. As I hit the gas and we

> sped out of town, I looked in the rear-view mirror: the young local guys were in a group, watching us leave. Call me suspicious, but I don't think they'd been following so they could invite us round for a cup of tea . . .

CHRIS RYAN'S STREET SAFETY DEBRIEF

- Train yourself to maintain a military level of situational awareness.
- Be hyper-aware of unusual signs and pre-incident indicators.
- Don't present yourself as a target.
- Take evasive action whenever possible.
- Never prioritise your belongings over your personal safety.
- If you have to use violence, ensure that it is effective.

4

STAYING SAFE IN YOUR CAR

SAS soldiers are good drivers. Rally-driver good. But they're not untouchable.

When I was in the Regiment, I was driving as part of a convoy through the Highlands of Scotland as part of the anti-terrorist team. Most of the unit was in Range Rovers, but part of the convoy was the MOE (Method of Entry) van.

The MOE van contained a massive amount of military equipment: not only door rams and hammers, but also high-explosives, shaped charges and detonators. On this occasion, it was overladen. The Regiment guy driving it had to scream the guts out of the engine to keep up with the Range Rover convoy along these steep, winding Highland roads.

We came to a bend. There was a ravine to the left. The Range Rovers took the corner, but the MOE van lost control. It left the road and rolled all the way down the hill. The driver and his passenger managed to get out and up the hill to safety. The vehicle itself was smouldering and smoking. We got the fire brigade out, but had to keep them back from the vehicle until we were sure there wouldn't be an explosion. If that thing had gone off, there would have been a hell of a bang.

On another occasion, I was driving back into Hereford after attending the bodyguarding course. I approached a bend and a Ford Escort suddenly emerged from a hidden exit up ahead. It was one of the 14 Int guys, who were doing high-speed chase training in the area. I swung immediately to the left, hit a ditch and flipped the vehicle. It landed on its roof. I had a dance track called 'Big Fun' blaring on the radio. It couldn't have been less appropriate!

Lots of Regiment guys died in their vehicles, and not always because of enemy action. It happened sometimes in Northern Ireland after an operation when they were returning to base, tired. A kid I put through selection tipped his Land Rover in Bosnia and died. And we had plenty of men killed in the Middle East in car crashes.

My point is this. Although SAS drivers find themselves in particularly hazardous driving scenarios, even the very best of them are subject to the dangers of the road. If you take one thing away from this chapter, let it be that it is very easy for people to overestimate their skillsets when it comes to driving. Cars are such everyday objects that we forget how dangerous they can be. Solid lumps of metal, driven at high speeds, often by people whose competence is not what it should be – no wonder that thousands of people die in motor vehicle collisions every year.

But these are not the only threats we face in our cars. Put road-rage incidents, vehicle thefts and carjackings into the mix, and it's pretty clear that the heightened level of awareness we apply in the streets is equally important when we're in, or near, our vehicles.

SAS VEHICLE SKILLS

SAS vehicle training is based around the fast-driving course. It's a bit of misnomer, because really it's a *safe*-driving course, although we are trained to maintain our safe-driving skills at speed, and while firing a weapon.

This is not something you'll need to do. However, there are elements of the SAS fast-driving course that will help keep you safe in everyday driving situations.

Understand your vehicle

It may not sound exciting, but this is the very first thing a Regiment driver is taught to do. I believe every civilian should make it a priority. Be honest: how many times have you jumped into a hire car at the airport without checking the location of all the controls you're going to need? This puts you at risk, because it means that at some point you're going to have to take your attention off the road while you find the indicators or the rear windscreen wipers. And it only takes a moment's inattention to cause a collision.

Every time you get into an unfamiliar vehicle, you should not only locate all the controls, you should sit behind the wheel, look straight ahead and make sure that you can locate them by touch alone. Even in a familiar vehicle, you should perform this exercise regularly.

You should always ensure that your seat is in the correct position so that you are sitting upright, can see further than the nose of the vehicle, and can comfortably have two hands on the steering wheel in the 10 and 2 o'clock positions. Forget the movie scenes where you see guys slouching at the wheel, turning it with a single finger, while burning down a country lane at 120 mph. Highly skilled motorists never drive that way.

Tyre pressures

The second thing SAS drivers are taught is the importance of tyre pressures. Most people only check their tyres every few months. Big mistake. Tyre pressure has a massive influence on a vehicle's handling and stopping. If a Regiment guy has to use a vehicle in an operational setting, it's unthinkable that he would let his tyres be under- or over-inflated if he could help it. On ops, we would check our tyre pressures every time we went out. In a civilian setting, once a week is a minimum requirement.

Vehicle equipment

There are certain items that I always carry in my vehicle:

- A head torch. If you need to change a tyre or put on snow chains in the dark, it's almost impossible without one of these.
- A hi-viz jacket. Roadsides are one of the least safe places you can find yourself. You need to be seen.
- A fire extinguisher.
- A tool kit.
- Snow chains. Spend five minutes learning how to put them on in dry conditions. Every year I see people trying to work them out in the Alps in horrendous weather. That's never going to end well.
- A warning triangle.

- A phone charger.
- A blanket.

Practise your observational skills

Just as we do it in the jungle, so we do it in our vehicles. It's the most important part of our fast-driving course. You go out with an instructor on to the road – it might be a motorway or a rural country lane – and you give a running commentary of everything you see up ahead and in your rear-view and side mirrors. You state out loud what's ahead of you or behind you. You observe that there's an entrance on the left-hand side, that you're travelling at 53 mph, that there's a major junction up ahead or a bend in 200 metres, so there's no chance of an overtake.

This is the vehicular equivalent of the heightened level of situational awareness I urged you to practise in the streets. It forces you to pay proper attention to the potential hazards all around you. It trains you not to lapse into the state of only semi-concentrating common to most drivers, and gives you a better chance of anticipating potential problems before they become actual problems.

You can practise this skill by yourself, of course, but it's one of the components of the advanced driving course, which I would recommend to anyone who wants to sharpen up their safe-driving skills.

In the previous chapter, we learned that it is impossible to maintain full situational awareness on the street when you're using your phone. This is doubly true when you're behind the wheel. Having your phone to your ear or – worse – texting while you're driving annihilates your situational awareness and your response times. It makes you oblivious to threats and unable to react to your environment. A trained driver would never do it. Nor should you.

Understand your limitations

SAS soldiers are taken on to a track and given instruction on handling vehicles at very high speeds. We learn how different vehicles react to high-speed manoeuvres and how to control them. These are not skills that most drivers will need. However, I think there is a benefit to regular drivers taking a vehicle out on a track, and it is this: you'll soon learn that your control over your vehicle is not as complete as you perhaps think it is.

As soon as a driver enters boy-racer mode, vehicle control is a whole new ball game. Serious drivers understand this. They understand that even professional rally drivers crash at speed. If you see someone burning down the road, far exceeding the safety limit, you can be quite sure that they are not a sophisticated, advanced driver. They are people who do not understand their own limitations, or the limitations of their vehicles.

EVASIVE DRIVING TECHNIQUES

Regiment guys are taught certain offensive and evasive driving techniques. Most of these involve weapons training and so are not appropriate to everyday driving situations, but there are some techniques that I believe might help a civilian in situations where their safety is under threat.

- When you come to a halt in a line of traffic, always make sure that you can see the rear wheels of the car in front of you. That way, if you get into trouble, you can pull out. If you can't see the wheels in front of you, you're boxed in.
- Avoid what my old regimental sergeant major called 'nosey parking' (we used to get fined if he saw us doing it). If you reverse park into a space, you can exit it much more quickly than if you forward park into it.
- Never let your fuel gauge dip below a quarter full. If you find yourself in a threatening situation, a quarter tank of fuel is enough to get you several tens of miles away, depending on your vehicle. Less than a quarter of a tank and you start compromising your ability to act evasively.

At the more extreme end of the scale, it can be useful to know the following three manoeuvres: the handbrake turn, the J-turn and the vehicle ram.

The handbrake turn

The scenario: you're driving along a road and up ahead you see a group of masked guys robbing a van. They're armed. You've got your family in the car. You need to turn round quickly. There are no other vehicles in your vicinity. If you can do a handbrake turn, you're out of there.

This manoeuvre will allow you to turn the car 180 degrees quickly and in a much tighter circle than the regular turning circle of a vehicle would allow. The vehicle will shift roughly its own width to the left or right, so there needs to be sufficient road width to do this.

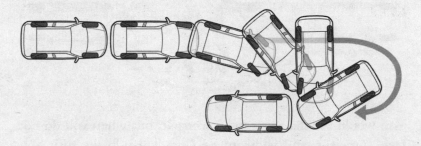

1. Position your car. When the nose is alongside the pivot point of the turn, you perform the manoeuvre.
2. Put your right hand across to the wrong side of the steering wheel – that is, to the 9 o'clock position (this is for a right-hand-drive car).
3. Put your left hand on the handbrake and press the button ready to engage it.
4. To make the turn, put as much clockwise steering lock on the vehicle as you can. Sharply engage the handbrake a fraction of a second after you turn the wheel. Don't be tempted to use the foot brake, but do engage the clutch as you pull the handbrake.
5. The car will spin. Turn your wheel so that your right hand moves back to the 9 o'clock position, so you know that your wheels are pointing straight ahead.
6. Release the handbrake and put yourself into first gear. Drive off safely.

The J-turn

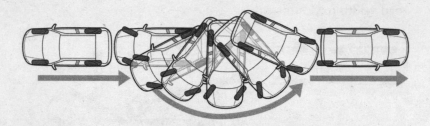

You would use this in a similar scenario, but when you do not have sufficient road width to perform a handbrake turn. You reverse away from the threat and perform the turn to get yourself driving in the same direction, but in forward gear. To do this (again in a right-hand-drive vehicle):

1. Put your vehicle into reverse.
2. Position your right hand at 9 o'clock on the steering wheel.
3. Either looking over your shoulder, or using your rear- and side-view mirrors, reverse to at least 20 mph, preferably nearer 40, in a straight line. This forces the weight of your vehicle on to the front tyres.
4. When you want to make the turn, release your foot from the accelerator and press down the clutch.
5. A fraction of a second after that, put full clockwise steering lock on the vehicle.
6. The car will spin. When it's moved through 90 degrees, move the steering wheel back to its original position with your hand at 9 o'clock and calmly put your transmission into second gear (or drive on an automatic).
7. Once you've completed the full 180, drive away.

These manoeuvres require practice: you should never try them in an on-road situation unless you're completely proficient. You need to find a race track or a disused runway to do this. Be careful, though: some runways have an anti-skid tarmac. A Regiment mate of mine was once practising handbrake turns on a runway in Northern Ireland and he flipped the car. Poor fella never heard the end of it!

The vehicle ram

You're approaching an offensive road block. A handbrake turn or J-turn is not practical. Your way is barred by one or two vehicles parked sideways. How do you break through?

First: forget the movies. It is possible to break through a road block, but not at the kind of speeds you see in films. If you try to ram another vehicle at fifty or sixty miles an hour, you'll probably kill yourself.

Equally, however, you do need a certain amount of speed to give your vehicle the correct momentum to bash the other car out of the way. The sweet spot is about 20 mph. If you are ramming a single vehicle aim for its rear wheels – engines are at the front, which means the back of the car is lighter and easier to shift. As you make contact, keep your foot on the accelerator to keep yourself powering through.

If two vehicles are blocking your way, you should still drive at 20 mph, but aim for the point where the two vehicles meet. Again, keep your foot on the accelerator as you make contact.

SECURING YOUR VEHICLE

There are hundreds of thousands of reported thefts from or of a car each year in the UK. You're never going to completely avoid opportunistic car crime. But there are things you can do to minimise the risk of this happening.

Modern vehicles have electronic anti-theft devices built in. These make them difficult to steal, but not impossible. It's common for car thieves to buy a new vehicle, strip it down and work out ways to bypass the security systems so that they can steal equivalent cars. Everything's hackable, so you shouldn't assume that just because you have the most up-to-date vehicle, it isn't going to be stolen. Keyless car theft is becoming a big problem, not least because the high-end vehicles that use electronic security systems are particularly prized by thieves, who steal them to order for distribution abroad. If you do have a vehicle with electronic security systems, you minimise your risk of car theft if you keep your vehicle software up to date, and be wary about connecting third-party devices to the diagnostics port.

However, hacking the vehicle security systems isn't the most common way of stealing a car. Most thieves don't have that kind of technical know-how. Their methods are more old-school, and so are the most effective countermeasures. (And if you don't have the most up-to-date Beemer, you're going to need to take some less hi-tech precautions anyway.)

Remember that there is never a shortage of potential vehicles to steal, and in general thieves are after the easiest target. If you take a few steps to make your vehicle a little bit tougher to swipe, a thief will most likely move on to simpler prey.

Hide your keys

As an SAS operative, I know that if I need to acquire a vehicle, the best way to do it is to break into a house that has a car in the drive and take the occupant's car keys. Criminals know this, too. A substantial proportion of car theft happens by thieves breaking and entering a house, then swiping the keys or the electronic fob. Why? Because most people come home and dump their car keys by the front door: fully on display, quick and easy to grab. A common trick is to use a fishing rod or pole through the letterbox. If you make a rigorous habit of hiding your keys, and of applying the home-security advice you'll find in the next chapter, you will make life ten times harder for the thief.

Switch your engine off

Never leave it running when you've left the vehicle – even if you're just nipping to the cash point. Vehicle thieves position themselves where this is likely to happen: outside supermarkets, petrol station forecourts, by fast-food restaurants. Don't walk into their trap.

Make your vehicle harder to tow

A common method of stealing a vehicle is simply to tow it away. Thieves do it brazenly, knowing that passers-by are likely to think they are attending a breakdown. There are a few simple things you can do to make your vehicle *much* harder to tow away.

- If you have a rear-wheel drive vehicle, park with the back of your vehicle close to a wall or stationary structure. If you have a front-wheel- or four-wheel-drive vehicle, do the same with the front of your vehicle.
- Always park with your wheels turned into the kerb – thieves will avoid towing it, because it will turn a full circle as they pull it away.
- Always engage your handbrake, and leave the vehicle in first gear if it's a manual transmission, or 'Park' if it's an automatic transmission.

Park in busy, well-lit areas

If you're parking during the day, but your vehicle is going to be unattended at night, think about what it will look like then. If I'm leaving my vehicle on the street, I always try to park under a street lamp, or outside a restaurant that I know will be busy come nightfall. It makes the car harder to steal, and means my own personal safety isn't compromised as I'm approaching it at night.

Fit a kill switch

Steering wheel locks are practically useless. They might serve as a bit of a deterrent, or act as the last line of defence in a car-theft scenario. But an experienced car thief can remove one of these in seconds with a chisel or a hammer and spike. Car alarms might also deter theft to a certain extent, but be honest: how many times have you heard one and ignored it?

The best vehicle security measure is to have an isolator switch fitted. These kill the flow of electricity to the battery or to the ignition switch, or they can disable the fuel pump. A decent mechanic will get one of these fitted up for you in an hour. Have the switch hidden somewhere in the vehicle only you know about. Even if they have your keys, or have hacked the electronics, or have tried to hotwire an older engine, that vehicle will never start. A thief isn't going to spend time trying to locate an isolator switch. Their priority is to get out of there quickly. They'll look for an easier target.

Avoid break-ins

Back in the day, car radios were prime targets for thieves. Not any more – they're cheap to buy, so have no resale value. Sat navs are a different matter. They have value and they're not registered to anyone. They should always be kept out of sight, but thieves aren't necessarily looking for the unit itself. They look for the telltale marking the sat-nav holder leaves on the windscreen. Make sure you wipe it off regularly.

If you have a sat nav in your vehicle, make sure it has a lock code, especially when you're out and about. Otherwise it's a moment's work to hit the home button and find your home address. If your car is parked in town, there's a good chance there's nobody at home, so your house is at a higher risk of a break-in.

Items of value should be taken with you or hidden from view in the boot. Thieves aren't stupid. Chucking your mobile under an old blanket is not good: messy cars are more likely to be broken into than tidy cars, because thieves know that people are lazy and hide their valuables under the debris in an untidy vehicle.

Fit a tracking device

Tracking devices are standard for vehicles used by the security services or special forces. But they're not only reserved for intelligence or military personnel. They're not cheap, and a tracking device won't stop your vehicle from being stolen. But if it is stolen, most vehicles with a tracking device are subsequently recovered (most without aren't).

CARJACKING

Carjacking is an effective way for thieves to thwart the countermeasures above: they steal the car while you're present. It can happen before you get into the car, while you're driving it, or when you get to your destination. It's a common crime, and if it happens to you, you're in a very dangerous situation. Carjacking might be committed by someone escaping a crime scene, by someone wanting to feed their drug habit, or even as a gang initiation. The bottom line is that the kind of person willing to carry out a carjacking is unlikely to have much respect for your personal safety, or even your life.

In order to avoid carjacking, you need to know the most common ways it's done.

- *The Bump*: The carjacker, with an associate in the passenger seat, bumps into the target vehicle from behind. The victim pulls over to check out the damage. Once he or she is no longer by the wheel, the carjacker takes the vehicle.
- *The 'Good Samaritan'*: The carjacker feigns an accident or

injury by the side of the road. The victim pulls over to help. The carjacker takes the vehicle.

- *The Worry Ruse*: The carjacker, with an associate in the passenger seat, pulls up behind the target vehicle and attracts their attention by flashing their lights and pointing at the target vehicle to indicate there's a problem. The two vehicles pull over, the victim gets out and the carjacking occurs.
- *The Follow Home*: The carjacker does just that. When the target vehicle comes to a halt and the victim emerges, the carjacking occurs.

There are certain locations where carjacking is more likely. These are:

- quiet, rural roads
- road intersections where you are obliged to stop
- high-crime areas
- empty car parks
- residential driveways
- traffic jams

As always, your first line of defence against a carjacking situation is heightened situational awareness. As you know by now, advanced drivers are trained to be more alert behind the wheel than normal drivers, but you should practise higher situational awareness when you approach your car and when you leave it, because these are statistically higher-risk moments.

While approaching your vehicle

As always, be alert for anyone who looks out of place or is showing any of the warning signs on pages 28–31. Be highly suspicious of anyone loitering in the vicinity of your vehicle – especially young males, particularly if they are ostentatiously asking for directions, handing out leaflets, or engaged in any activity that might just be a cover story for their presence. Trust your instincts.

Have your car key ready well in advance of approaching your parked car, so you can get in immediately rather than hanging around hunting for your keys and making yourself a target. (In an operational setting, I would always carry my keys in my non-dominant hand, so that my dominant hand is available for self-defence if the situation requires it. If I felt threatened, I would have my key hand in a fist shape, with the key itself sticking out from between my fingers.)

When you enter your car, lock your doors and get moving as quickly as possible. Too many people sit behind the wheel, looking in their handbag, checking their phone, maybe making a call. This is a prime opportunity for a carjacker or thief to hit an unsuspecting driver. Their situational awareness is momentarily lowered, because they think they're safe in their car. They're not.

While driving

Keep your vehicle doors locked and your windows up. Do this even if you're only travelling a short distance.

On slow roads, drive in the inside or centre lane. This puts you less at risk of carjacking by people waiting at the side of the road. Driving in the centre lane also makes it harder for other vehicles to box you in.

As mentioned above, when you come to a halt in a line of traffic, always make sure you can see the back wheels of the vehicle in front of you. This ensures that you have sufficient space to manoeuvre round the car if you feel threatened in any way.

If someone drives into the back of you, don't stop immediately. Make a mental note of the car's registration number and indicate to them that they should follow. Drive to a safe, well-lit, busy location of your choosing before you risk pulling over and making contact. Alternatively, stay in the vehicle with your doors locked and the windows up, and call the police.

Think twice before stopping to help a stranger whose car appears to have broken down on the side of the road. If you want to give assistance, drive on a bit and call the police for help.

When you reach your destination

Park tactically. If possible, park near other vehicles, in a well-lit, busy area near the entrance of your destination. In an operational setting, I would always do a full circuit of a parking area to scope it out for threats before parking.

Avoid parking near areas that give criminals cover, such as large lorries or heavy foliage.

Check your mirrors for potential threats before unlocking your car doors and stepping outside.

If, despite all these precautions, somebody attempts to carjack you, make no mistake that you are in an extremely dangerous situation. The carjacker will most likely be on edge and all the advice I gave you in the previous chapter about prioritising your life over your possessions still holds. You should let them take the car, your wallet, your valuables, whatever they want – but with two caveats.

Firstly, if you have a child in the car, the carjacker may not have seen them. You need to make them *very* aware of the child's presence. Most carjackers only want the vehicle – not the added complication of an abducted child.

Secondly, you should never agree to go anywhere *with* the carjacker, if you can possibly prevent it. This turns a carjacking into a hostage situation, which is much more serious. Later in the book, I'll explain more about your best response to a hostage situation. But if you're forced to drive in a carjacking situation, consider crashing the car when it's safe to do so – preferably somewhere busy, but obviously where you're not going to injure anybody else. Then get out of the car and run.

French motorways are a real hotspot for carjackings. It was on one of these that somebody tried it on with me.

My ferry from the UK had been diverted. It put a couple of hours on the journey through France and meant I hit the motorway at night. I felt myself nodding off at the wheel, so I pulled into a rest area, where I parked opposite the well-lit toilet block. I killed the ignition but, in my tiredness, made the error of not locking my doors before immediately falling asleep.

I don't think I'd been asleep for more than a couple of minutes before I sensed that there was someone approaching the vehicle. As I opened my eyes, I saw a figure walking round the front of the car toward the driver's door. Before I knew what was happening, he was trying to open it. I then realised a second guy had approached the passenger seat. I reckon they'd been planning to wait for me to leave the vehicle. If I'd left it unlocked, they'd have jumped in and stolen it. When it was clear that I was staying put, they'd decided to try the direct result.

I quickly started the engine and pulled forward about ten feet before they could gain access to the vehicle. Then I stopped. I'm sorry to say that I failed to follow the advice I'm giving you in this book, which would be to get out of there as quickly as possible. I knocked the vehicle into reverse and sped back to where these two thugs were still standing, planning to confront them. Seriously: don't do this. Not only do you risk exposing yourself to a fight you don't want, you also risk scratching your motor when your wannabe carjacker bounces off the side. (I speak from experience!)

HOW TO CHECK IF YOU'RE BEING FOLLOWED IN A VEHICLE

Professional surveillance personnel are extremely adept at following targets without being noticed. They work in tandem with other vehicles, so their target doesn't become suspicious of a single vehicle on their tail. They know what distance to keep and have strategies for dealing with any counter-surveillance moves you might have up your sleeve. The bottom line is that if you're being followed by a pro, you won't know about it unless you've been trained.

But you probably *aren't* being followed by a pro. Carjackers, stalkers and thieves won't have these skills. So there are two simple techniques that will help you establish whether you really are being followed, or if you're mistaken.

Keep turning

If you're in an urban environment, take a sequence of four right or four left turns. If possible, do this so you end up back on the road where you started. The likelihood of a random driver spontaneously doing the same is practically zero.

If you can't make this pattern, simply make a zigzagging sequence of left and right turns. If the vehicle is still in sight after six or seven of these, it's tailing you.

Alternatively, take a few spins round a roundabout. If the car behind does the same, it's following.

Make tactical use of motorway exits

If you're on the motorway, pull off at the next exit, but then get straight back on to the motorway. Car still in your rear-view mirror? You're being followed.

WHAT TO DO IF YOU'RE BEING FOLLOWED BY A VEHICLE

First off, try to keep calm. Being followed is scary, but you don't want to let your anxiety compromise your driving skills.

Don't keep looking in the rear-view mirror. People often crash in this situation, because they're focusing more on what's behind them than on what's in front of them. You've confirmed you're being followed – you don't need to keep reconfirming it.

I'm hoping that your vehicle doors are already locked. If they aren't: lock them.

If you can safely make a mobile-phone call, call the police. Tell them your location and your registration number. Give a description of the car following you and, if possible, its registration number. If you're a lone female, or have children in the vehicle, make that clear.

If possible, drive to a police station. Park up outside it, but don't exit the vehicle or unlock the doors. You'll probably find that your tail doesn't want to discuss his or her presence with the local police.

Avoid empty, rural lanes.

Don't drive home. Hopefully the person following you doesn't know your home address. Let's keep it that way.

In general, you should stick to busy areas. However, if you can get on to a motorway, you can take a leaf out of the book of the Russian mafia, who have a technique of meeting on the motorway hard shoulder, so that any covert surveillance has to keep travelling past them. If you pull over on the hard shoulder, the person following will be forced to continue past you if they don't want to reveal themselves. (I should point out that this does *not* conform to the rules of the road. Mis-using the hard shoulder can be fatal. This is an emergency situation manoeuvre only.)

HOW TO DEAL WITH ROAD RAGE AND AGGRESSIVE DRIVERS

Driving can be stressful, and road rage is common even in people who are normally in control of their emotions. So, our first priority when it comes to avoiding road rage is to take steps not to allow ourselves to succumb to it.

SAS operatives put themselves in stressful environments often. In order to stay safe, they need to apply certain positive psychological techniques to keep control of their instinctive aggression, so that they avoid putting themselves in unnecessary danger. We can use some of these techniques in our vehicles to ensure that we're not the ones who allow a conflict situation to escalate:

- Understand that, when we succumb to road rage, other road users are merely a stimulus for our own frustration. We can take steps to calm that frustration before we get into our vehicle. Leave in good time. Make sure you're comfortable.

- Accept that a proportion of other road users may be stupid, thoughtless or incompetent. This is not news to you, and you're not going to change it. Their stupidity is not your problem. Your safety is.
- Consider what the consequences will be for you if you lose yourself to road rage. Lose your job? A fine? Prison?
- Remember that, no matter how big or tough you are, conflict situations are unpredictable. Do you really want to bang on someone's window to give him some aggro, only to find he's got a screwdriver in his pocket?

Now we need to think about how to avoid road rage in others:

- Don't drive aggressively yourself. If you cut someone up, or start honking at them, you risk sparking a road-rage incident.
- Avoid eye contact with aggressive drivers. They may see it as a challenge.
- Don't react to aggressive manoeuvres. If someone honks you, don't honk them back. If someone cuts you up, don't do the same to them.
- Give right of way to aggressive drivers. It doesn't matter that you're in the right and they're in the wrong. Swallow your pride. Be the grey man (or woman).
- If an aggressive driver starts following you, see the advice on page 71. Especially, do not drive home: you don't want an enraged driver following you there. If you're on a main road, drive off at the next exit. Road rage is not premeditated. An enraged driver probably has somewhere to be, so they're unlikely to follow you very far out of their way.

If an enraged driver gets out of their vehicle and approaches yours when you're at a standstill, you're entering a potentially deadly situation. If you can drive away, do that. If not:

- Make sure your doors are locked and your windows closed. Despite what you see in the movies, it's incredibly difficult to break car windows with your fists, so inside the vehicle is the safest place to be. Do not get out of your car.
- Call the police. At the very least, put your phone to your ear to make it *look* as if you're doing so.
- Make a lot of commotion. Honk your horn, flash your lights. Make use of the fact that your aggressor probably doesn't want to become the centre of attention.

If for any reason you are forced out of your vehicle, your first priority must be to run if you can safely do so. If you can't, you need to defend yourself and to strike pre-emptively and effectively if it is appropriate. See Chapter Eleven for more on this.

SAT NAVS

We all have them, and we know how useful they are. But I want you to remember what I explained about positional awareness in the jungle. Knowing where we are, and how to get to where we want to be, is an essential component of our personal security. For this reason, I would never have blind faith in my sat nav. I always back it up with a road atlas, so that I can double-check the route I'm taking to make sure, a) it's the most efficient route, b) it doesn't take me through dodgy areas where I don't want to find myself and c) it is suitable for the vehicle I'm driving. I also want to be sure that I know where I am at all points along that route.

Too many drivers cede the decision-making process to the sat nav. Don't be seduced into thinking you can get away with being less aware, just because the box is talking to you. GPS was developed for the military, but a good soldier would never trust the machine over his or her senses, any more than they would trust a weapon to kill an enemy target by itself. It's a tool, nothing more.

Remember: you're the one driving, not the sat nav. Your eyes and general situational awareness are more powerful than its circuitry. Your eyes should always be on the road, not on the screen. And, as with mobile phones, never try to program it while you're driving.

DASH CAMS

In war zones, many modern soldiers wear helmet cams. Special forces soldiers utilise them to relay footage back to their controllers, but most green army guys use them as personal insurance: they provide documentary proof that they're acting lawfully on the battlefield.

Dash cams serve a similar purpose for the civilian driver. They record on a constant loop as soon as the car starts up. If there's a dispute over a motor-vehicle collision, they can provide evidence that you're not at fault. They are also a powerful tool for countering 'crash-for-cash' scams (see pages 123–4 for more on these). But for my money, they have a more significant role: carjackers and enraged drivers are much less likely to engage in violent activity if they spot a dash cam on your windscreen. They are a very effective personal security tool.

Some dash cams have two cameras: one to film the front, one to film the back. This is the type I'd recommend.

The principal message of this chapter is one of avoidance and de-escalation. I wouldn't ordinarily recommend that a vehicle be used offensively in a civilian scenario. But I'd never say never.

In 2013, a guy who I'll call Jack – again not his real name – was driving through a major city with his wife and daughter. He found himself surrounded by a group of bikers, who were taking part in an annual street ride. They were driving aggressively. One of the bikers cut across Jack's vehicle and slowed down, causing Jack to clip him with his bumper.

The shit hit the fan. The bikers surrounded Jack's vehicle and started to slash his tyres. Fearing for the safety of his family, Jack tried to escape, but hit three of the bikers in the process. The bikers chased him and, when he became caught up in traffic, they surrounded his vehicle again. One of the bikers used his motorbike helmet as a tool to smash the driver's window. They pulled Jack from the car and started to lay into him, again using their helmets as weapons. He was knocked unconscious.

It was only because an onlooker begged the bikers to leave Jack's family alone that his wife and daughter were unharmed. The bikers sped away from the scene. Jack was taken to hospital where he received stitches to the face and treatment for a badly beaten torso.

Jack had done very little wrong. A scenario like this goes to show how our safety can be compromised when we least expect it and through no fault of our own. This, however, is how I would have handled the situation.

While driving, I would have taken pains to be hyper-aware of what was happening on the road at least fifty metres up ahead. If I became aware of any kind of unusual driving conditions – and a crowd of bikers would certainly fall into this category – I would immediately take evasive action. Pull over, if possible. Turn round. Take another route. Don't worry about being overcautious. Caution is the watchword of the special forces operative.

If, however, it was becoming apparent that I couldn't avoid the bikers, I would immediately check that all the car doors were locked and the windows up. If there was a person in the passenger seat, as there was on this occasion, I would have them grab the road map and immediately search for a main thoroughfare out of the immediate vicinity. I would probably not rely on my sat nav unless there was no other option, because I wouldn't be in control of the route it suggested: I wouldn't want it taking me down slow, narrow streets, where I could easily be stopped or boxed in by aggressive bikers.

Once it became clear that the bikers were surrounding me and acting aggressively, I would have my passenger call the police. The very moment it became apparent that my safety or that of my family was under threat, my priority would be to remove myself from the situation. If I could get out of there by performing a J-turn, I would do that. Otherwise, I would have no hesitation in using my vehicle offensively. I wouldn't worry about damaging it. Always: personal safety above possessions. If a motor-bike was blocking my way, I would aim for its front or rear wheel rather than hitting it fully side on, as this would make it more likely to spin out of my way. If my path was still blocked, I would reverse hard and go again.

If the bikers were using their helmets to break my car windows, I would do everything in my power not to let them get any closer to me or my family. The broken window would provide me with a very effective weapon: glass shards. I would use these to fight back as aggressively as possible, making it very clear that I was not an easy target. Violence, when you use it, has to be effective.

Once I was free of the biker mob, I would prioritise getting myself on to a main arterial road. I would understand that I have no chance of outrunning a motorbike, and that I need to keep moving. I would drive as close as I could to one side of the road (if I was on a motorway I would stick in the fast lane), so that I couldn't be boxed in on both sides. This tactic would mitigate their numerical advantage to a certain extent. And while I would not recommend that this is something you should do, I'm clear in my own mind that if a motorbike tried to slow me down by riding in front of me, and was threatening my family by doing so, I'd knock him off his bike.

All the while, I or my passenger would be on the phone to the police, explaining what was going on and keeping them constantly updated with my location. On no account would I stop if I could help it, because I know that I'd come out worse in an unarmed fight against that number of people.

CHRIS RYAN'S VEHICLE SAFETY DEBRIEF

- Understanding your vehicle is important. Understanding your own limitations as a driver, even more so.
- The main difference between a pro driver and a regular driver is a heightened level of awareness and an ability to spot threats well in advance.
- The most effective vehicle-security measure is a hidden isolator switch.
- Carjackings are more common than you think. Be suspicious of any attempt to get you to stop your vehicle. If someone bumps into you, don't just pull over there and then.
- Take unlikely routes to establish whether you're being followed. If you are: stay calm, stick to busy areas and don't drive home. Call the police.
- Don't rely on sat navs. Do rely on dash cams.

5

STAYING SAFE IN YOUR HOME

I had a mate in the Regiment who was a heavy drinker. He walked into camp one morning, his face swollen and bleeding. This didn't happen often. Mostly, if one of the SAS guys got into a fight with the pointy-heads (our name for the Hereford locals), it was the pointy-heads who came off worse. So obviously everyone wanted to know what had happened.

Sure enough, this fella had gone out on the lash in Hereford. Ten pints later, he'd arrived back home to find that his missus had changed the locks on the door. Always one to take the direct approach, he'd kicked the door in. Easy. He staggered into the kitchen and started rummaging through the cupboards looking for something to eat to soak up the booze. But his wife had changed all the cupboards around and in his drunken stupor he couldn't find anything to eat. Eventually he managed to put his hands on a box of cornflakes. He poured himself a bowl, slapped it down on the kitchen table and started to eat.

The next thing he knew, he was being whacked over the head and in the face with an iron bar.

He hit the ground – a drunken, unconscious, bleeding mess. It was only when he woke up that he realised he was in the wrong house. He'd kicked in his neighbour's door. When the neighbour had seen this broad-shouldered, steaming SAS man guzzling cornflakes at her kitchen table, she'd taken steps to defend herself. Nothing wrong with that – but my mate was a bit more careful about breaking down random doors in Hereford from then on . . .

Generally speaking, your house is safe from drunken SAS men. However, although we all like to feel secure in our own homes, the brutal truth is that we're not necessarily. There are approximately 750,000 instances of domestic burglary in the UK every year. When an incident like this happens and you're in the house, your personal safety is clearly threatened. You need to be aware of that threat. Vigilance is necessary, even within the four walls of your house.

There are limits, of course. When I was first dating my wife, she was a theatre sister in the army, coordinating all the equipment and instruments in the operating theatre. I was staying with her on one occasion. She went off to work and I went out for a run. I got back, showered and was in the bathroom shaving. Suddenly, unexpectedly, I saw the bathroom door move. I acted without even thinking – it was my Regiment training instinctively kicking in – and thumped the door back with my heel as hard as I could. It was my wife. The sharp edge of the door, and the force of my kick, split her face right open. She's never let me forget it!

An SAS man doesn't like being snuck up on. The heightened level of awareness that we maintain at work sticks with us, even when we're in the safety of our own four walls. On ops, it keeps us alive. At home, it can be a problem. A lot of the guys find, especially after a long tour, that when they get home they are overly sensitive to ordinary goings on in the house. More than once, I'd be dozing in a chair and my young daughter would creep up on me, only to find herself suddenly grabbed and shouted at. Frightening for her, hurtful for me – it usually ended up with both of us crying.

So, I don't want to make you think that you need to turn your house into a fortress, or to pretend that your home is some sort of war zone. Later in this chapter, I will encourage you to think about how you might act if an intruder enters while you're at home, but first I want to encourage you to take some fairly simple security precautions. Like my mate with the black eye, I could break into your house in a matter of seconds. And if I can do it, so can other people. Your job is to make it hard for them.

THINK LIKE A THIEF (OR AN SAS SOLDIER)

Just like muggers and car thieves, burglars and home intruders want an easy life. They don't home in on potentially difficult targets. They want easy pickings. When it comes to burglary, that means houses that they can access easily and without being seen.

Consequently, they have the same mindset, if not the same skillset, as an SAS soldier. If we were to put in surveillance on a target's house with the intention of breaking in, we would look for its weak points. Is there an area of shadow in the garden we can use to make an approach? Which door appears to be the weakest? What time does the target generally leave and return? Is there an intruder alarm? Armed with this kind of intel, we can be in and out quietly and quickly and with nobody the wiser.

That's what a burglar wants to do. To make it tough for him, you need to think like a thief. Walk down your street and imagine you were a burglar casing the area, looking for a likely house to hit. Is it going to be the one with the security gates, burglar alarm and dog bowl on the front step? Or is it going to be the one with untouched letters protruding from the letter box, and a window at the side swinging open?

The answer is obvious, but often we don't see it. We're hard-wired to accept our environment as being 'normal' and to believe the fallacy that, since we haven't been burgled yet, it's unlikely to happen. Thieves (and undercover operatives) take advantage of this.

Now, once you've carried out your neighbourhood surveillance, return to your own house. Having identified the weak points in other houses, I'm hoping you'll be able to look at your home through fresh eyes.

BURGLAR-PROOFING YOUR HOUSE

Back in the early eighties, some of the SAS lads used to travel across the pond to work on method-of-entry techniques with the LAPD. The American cops had a big problem at the time breaking into crack houses. The dealers would line the interior of their houses with sheet metal and install metal frames around the doors. It made them practically impregnable. The only way the LAPD could break in, other than using explosive charges, was to fit ramrods to military-grade vehicles. These ramrods had special spikes on the end. Once they broke through a steel-plated door, the rods would open up so that when the vehicle reversed, it would rip the whole doorframe out.

I'm not suggesting that you should make like an LA crack dealer and wallpaper your house with sheet metal. But there are some simple, effective measures you can take to ensure that your house is less likely to be burgled or broken into.

Brace your doors

Most break-ins are not sophisticated. Like my drunk mate, a burglar will often simply kick your door in. They know which doors are easy to break down and which aren't. So should you.

If a door only has a single cylinder lock (like a Yale lock), it's easy to break in. I could pick a lock like that in seconds and kick the door down in not much longer. Trust me: it's a thief magnet.

Most people advise that you have at least a second mortise deadlock fitted to your front door. Personally, I've seen too many of those opened without much trouble. In order to make a door almost impregnable to an opportunistic burglar, I'd suggest the following additional precautions. I know that these would make it much harder for me to break down a door:

- Make sure every exterior door is solid, with no weak panels and no glazing.
- Reinforce your strike plate. This is the metal panel on your door frame that your bolts slide into. Most strike plates are

insubstantial and only attached with short screws. This is what makes many doors so easy to kick in. At the very least, you should upgrade the screws so they are at least two inches long. Better, fit a burglar-proof strike plate – these are long metal strips that can be screwed into the door frame at multiple points, making the door far harder to kick in.

- Fit extra deadbolts opposite the hinges of the door. The extra security at the top and bottom of the door make it almost impossible to rip out of the frame.

Always ensure that your door *looks* like it's in good nick. If it's tatty, burglars might assume that it's old, uncared for and insecure, which will make them more likely to give your house a try.

Secure your windows

All windows should have window locks to stop them opening fully. This goes for first-floor windows, too – don't fool yourself that a thief can't access them easily.

Most thieves will avoid breaking windows, because of the noise it makes, but I would always recommend toughened glass to make it that bit more difficult for them.

Lighting

Lots of burglaries happen during the day when the occupants of the house are out at work. But many burglars still prefer the cover of darkness. Bright lights, at night, will always deter them. Movement-operated security lights do the job well. I always make certain that my house is surrounded by them. If somebody who wants to do you harm has performed surveillance on your house, they will have taken note of any spots in the garden or surrounding area that aren't covered by security lights. Remember: burglars don't want to be seen by the neighbours any more than they want to be seen by you. If possible, make sure the approaches to your house are also lit up when viewed from the street.

LED lights are very cost efficient – you can place fifteen lights around your house and use the same amount of power as single halogen security light.

People often recommend putting an interior light on a timer when you're out of the house. I would suggest using several, set to come on at different times. If an intruder is conducting surveillance on your house, they'll soon notice that a single light is coming on at the same time. It's more difficult to keep track of many different lights.

Cover

Cover is a lifeline to a burglar, just as it is to a soldier. Don't provide it to them. You might feel more private and secure if your house is surrounded by tall trees and bushes, but in reality you're playing into a burglar's hands by giving them an easy place to hide, and a barrier to stop neighbours seeing them break into your house. High 'privacy' fences might look like a good security measure, but they are easy to scale and offer perfect cover from neighbours.

Defensive plants

None of us want razor wire over our fences. A time-honoured and extremely effective alternative is to use spiny or prickly plants. Rambling roses growing up and over a wall will prevent an intruder just as effectively as barbed wire. A thicket of prickly shrubs will stop a potential burglar from crossing open ground. Defensive plants are particularly effective when grown around windows as these can be easy access points. My go-to defensive plant is *Pyracantha*. It has long, extremely sharp thorns and can be pruned into a box shape under windows so that it looks attractive. It will deter any intruder.

Grease

Drainpipes – especially solid cast iron ones – offer easy access to first-floor windows. An old SAS trick is to smear grease over the drainpipes, which makes them incredibly difficult to shimmy up. They also mark your intruder with grease to make a subsequent arrest more likely.

Line of sight

If I'm setting up a defensive position – and in some ways that's what your house is – I want to make sure I have full line of sight over all approaches to it. If I don't, I need some other way of alerting myself to an approach from that aspect, and of defending that line of attack. In a domestic setting, this means that any area of the garden that I can't see from my house needs extra attention with respect to lighting, cover and defensive plants.

Burglar alarms

I wouldn't bother with fake alarm fascias, or stickers announcing security measures that don't exist. Burglars can spot them a mile off. If you're going to get an alarm (and I think you should), get a good quality one with a brand name that a potential burglar will recognise and therefore avoid.

Regular alarms that make a loud noise when someone opens a door or breaks a window can be a good deterrent. Even better is a full home security system – the type that contacts an external security contractor if it's triggered. These can be expensive, though, and they're not foolproof. A common scam involves getting a job at the alarm company and hiring out your services to criminals who want to bypass the alarms.

By far the best alarm is a dog. There's no two ways about it. When a criminal hears a dog barking, they won't know if it's a pitbull or a poodle, so they probably won't risk an encounter. But the main reason a dog is so effective is that the noise of barking potentially alerts people to an intruder's presence.

Even if you don't have a dog, keeping a dog bowl by your front and back door is a very effective burglary countermeasure.

Gravel

Simple but effective: gravel around the house makes it very hard for an intruder to approach without being heard. If they see it, they'll tend to go for a softer target.

Secure your garaging

If I wanted to break into a target's house, I'd head for the garage or shed first, if there is one. They are often full of tools that make it easy to break into a house. Always make sure your garage is locked. Especially, padlock any ladders to a fixed point so they can't be used to get into first- or second-floor windows.

Tidy up

You can tell a lot about a house simply by looking at its immediate surroundings:

- Are there teenagers' bikes in the garden? That means there's likely to be a valuable games console inside (not to mention that a bike could easily be used to break a window).
- Are there kids' toys lying around? Kids normally mean mums, and mums often mean jewellery.
- Does the lawn need mowing? That suggests nobody's been around for a while.
- Are there leaflets on the doormat, or even protruding from the letterbox? Ditto.

A common trick to tell if somebody is on holiday is for an intruder to put a leaflet in the letterbox themselves. If it's still there the next day, that's telling you something. So if you do go away, get a neighbour to collect your post for you every day.

WHO ARE YOU LETTING INTO YOUR HOME?

If you engage contractors, always vet them thoroughly and ask for references. If someone comes to your door wanting to read a meter or talk to you about home repairs, ask them to return at a prearranged time. A common burglary technique is to gain access to someone's home with their permission and survey the place from the inside. It's even common for contractors to unlock a door or window so they can gain easy access later. Don't be fooled by their charm.

Bottom line: I would always view an unknown, unvetted visitor to my house with caution.

ANSWERING YOUR DOOR

First things first: your front door should have a peep-hole, so you can see who is on the other side. Forget about those security chains that allow you to open the door a few inches to see who's there. As soon as the door is open, an intruder can barge it and the security chain will snap like a twig.

It can be tempting, if you don't recognise the person at the door, or are not expecting anyone to call, to ignore them and pretend you're not home. *This is a very bad idea.* One of the first things an intruder will do is ring the doorbell or knock on the door. If there's no response, that's an indication that this is a good house to break into.

If there is somebody at the door, tell them loudly and confidently that you don't answer to unexpected guests. If they are persistent, state that you are immediately calling the police. They'll soon leave.

Dressing up as a delivery man is a common tactic, both of security-service personnel and intruders. Delivery guys seldom look out of place, and people readily open the door to them. So only open the door to a delivery person if you're expecting a delivery. If you're not sure, ask for the delivery guy's details and call the delivery service to confirm their identity.

THE DOUBLE CAMERA TRICK

A set of CCTV cameras is a very effective security measure (although you should be aware that it may indicate that there is something in your house worth stealing). An even better security measure – and this is a common SAS trick – is *two* sets of security cameras. One on display, one covert. Intruders sometimes manage to disable or dodge security cameras. But if they've done one set, they generally won't think to look for a second. That's how you catch them.

When I was in the Regiment, we had a fruit machine in the sergeant's mess. There came a time when the lads would turn up every morning to find that the machine had been broken into and the money inside stolen. A couple of us set up a trap. We rigged a camera, but it had an obvious blind spot. At the same time, we rigged a covert camera that would give us a good view of the fruit machine and whoever was breaking into it. Sure enough, our guy worked out how to approach the fruit machine without being viewed on the overt camera, but we caught him red-handed breaking into the fruit machine on the covert camera. He was only attached to the Regiment, rather than being one of the regular guys, so he wasn't wise to our scheme.

Obviously, a covert camera won't stop a break-in, but it may give you the evidence you need to catch your thief and regain your possessions.

BE CAREFUL WHAT GOES IN YOUR RUBBISH BIN

For people who are planning to burgle you or do you harm, information is gold dust. Don't hand it to them. If you put sensitive documents into your outdoor rubbish bin, that's what you're doing.

I'd recommend investing in a shredder and destroying all documents that contain personal information (for example, your name, telephone number, bank details and insurance details) before throwing them away.

But it's not only what's *in* your rubbish bin that matters. If you've just bought a new fancy computer or flat-screen TV and the empty box is propped up by your bins waiting for collections, it's a beacon to a thief, because it tells them there's something worth robbing here. Much better to cut the box up into little bits. Better still, take it to the dump immediately.

HIDING VALUABLES

Thieves want an easy ride. But once they've gone to the trouble of getting into your house, they're unlikely to leave until they have something of value to show for it.

This means that they will spend time looking for valuables. Hiding your jewellery in your underwear drawer – or in any other obvious places – is clearly a bad idea. If you search the internet for crafty places to hide your valuables, you'll come up with lots of seemingly clever ideas (wrapped in tinfoil in the freezer, shoved into cereal packets at the back of the cupboard, in your toilet cistern). Trust me: burglars have seen it all before. This is their job, and they're good at it. You won't fool them.

The only truly safe place to hide your valuables at home is in a sturdy safe that has been bolted to the floor. By all means put the safe in a difficult-to-find, inaccessible place, but your first line of defence is that these are impregnable to a regular thief, and can't be taken away. You can also get fireproof safes that protect your valuables in the event of a fire.

Think carefully about what is genuinely valuable. Most people focus on jewellery and cash. In fact, passports and other identifying documents (such as mortgage papers and insurance certificates) are just as valuable, because they can be sold on for identity fraud, which is a very big criminal business.

DECOY VALUABLES

Military tacticians often make use of a decoy. If a Regiment unit is planning to hit a target from one direction, it's common practice to arrange a decoy hit from another direction in order to divert the target's attention.

It is effective to use a similar tactic in your home. A burglar is likely to leave your house once they have something of value. Keeping some paper currency in a location they are likely to search (like a sock drawer or jewellery box – most burglars head straight for the master bedroom) can be an effective decoy.

Many burglars will be pleased to have stolen *something*, and will prioritise exiting safely over going for a bigger prize.

WHAT TO DO IF AN INTRUDER GETS INTO YOUR HOUSE

If an intruder gets into your house while you are still there, you'll be frightened. So you should be. This is a potentially lethal situation. Either the intruder has gained access to the house with the specific intention of doing you harm, or they will be on-edge burglars, and volatile. They may very well be armed.

For these reasons, it is a good idea to have a dedicated safe room in your house.

Safe rooms

If I was bodyguarding somebody in a house, one of the first things I would establish would be a safe room. At its most basic, it would simply be a room with a lock on the door where I could incarcerate my principal if there was an intruder. However, we can do a bit better than that.

A safe room should be located where everyone in the house can easily get to it at night. A first-floor bedroom with an en-suite shower room would be perfect: close to the other bedrooms, it has sanitation facilities and no ground-floor windows to provide an easy alternative access point for an intruder.

Interior doors are far easier to break down than exterior doors. I would always try to fit an exterior door to a safe room, and apply the same care to its locking mechanisms as noted above. I would also reinforce the strike plate, as above.

If my safe room had to be on the ground floor, I would try to make it in a room that has no exterior windows. If I couldn't do that, I would ensure that any external windows had toughened glass and heavy curtains to make access more difficult and to stop yourself from being seen.

One of those wedge-shaped door jams is a very effective tool for stopping somebody from entering a room – I don't care who they are, they'll have trouble kicking in a door that is stoppered with one of them on the inside.

Perhaps the most important element of the safe room, however, would be a phone. Use an old mobile handset with a pay-as-you-go SIM card, and keep it permanently plugged in *inside* your safe room. This means that you can dial 999 as soon as you're inside. If you do this, maintain an open line so that you can keep the emergency services informed of what is happening. This is important for their safety if they arrive to find an armed intruder, but it's important for yours, too. In a later chapter, you'll learn that one of the most dangerous moments in a hostage situation is when help arrives, because it can be hard for the responders to know who are the good guys and who are the bad guys. Same here. If you can keep the police aware of your location, you can make sure there are no mix-ups.

I would keep a solid weapon, such as a baseball bat, in my safe room, in the event that I need to defend myself (see below).

A safe room is not a bunker where you'll be spending days on end. You don't need to worry about stocking it with food or other supplies. You'll hopefully only be in there for as long as it takes for the police to arrive. However, you *mustn't* leave until you're completely sure it's safe to do so. Don't be fooled by an intruder going quiet on you. You need confirmation that the police are on site and the house is secure.

Establishing a safe room might sound a bit extreme, but it's certainly a good idea if you live in an area where there are a lot of burglaries. And even if you don't live in such an area, a basic safe room is – as I mentioned above – simply a room with a lock that you can operate from the inside. Not a big deal for a simple security measure.

Action plans

In order for a safe room to be effective, everybody in your family needs to be aware of it. They need to know what to do in the event of there being an intruder. Make sure all your family know how to get there in the dark. Above all, practise doing it. At the beginning of this section, I made the point that this is a very frightening situation. When we're frightened, our ability to think and act clearly can be compromised. The reason soldiers practise their combat routines so thoroughly is in order that these routines should become second nature when they are under stress and under fire. If you have an intruder in your house, you're definitely under stress and you *might* be under fire. Take a leaf out of the soldier's manual and practise your evasive manoeuvres. Do some night-time safe-room drills with your family.

Keeping quiet vs making a noise

The decision whether to make a noise or to keep quiet will be determined by the circumstances. If you're locking yourself in a safe room and you believe that the intruder is not aware of your presence or your movements, you should keep quiet so they can't pinpoint your position.

If you're face to face with the intruder, or they're trying to break in to your safe room or hiding place, you'll have to make a call about how much noise to make. If you just want them to take what they want and then leave, keep calm. If you sense that you're in a potential conflict situation, I would make as much noise as possible and yell at your intruder that the police are on their way. If you have neighbours, shouting from a window to raise the alarm might be the right call. If you have a smoke alarm (and you should), they mostly have a test button on the underside. Engaging this and keeping it down will make enough noise to scare off most intruders.

In either scenario, if you have a car key fob that can remotely set off your car alarm, use it – the noise will probably encourage an intruder to leave.

Blockading

Doors are very difficult to open if they've been blockaded. If you're under threat, you can barricade yourself into a safe room – or indeed any room – by dragging a chest of drawers or a heavy piece of furniture across the door. I would recommend this particularly if you think your intruder might be armed. Combined with the wedge-shaped door jam (above), you'll make it very difficult for an attacker to gain access.

If you blockade the door, don't let it lull you into a false sense of security. Don't stand in front of the blockade (you'll be in the line of fire if your intruder has a firearm) and especially don't stand close to the door – if your intruder manages to stick a knife or screwdriver through door, you'll risk being hit.

YOU HEAR A NOISE DOWNSTAIRS AT NIGHT. YOU'RE NOT SURE IT'S AN INTRUDER. WHAT DO YOU DO?

Realistically, you're going to have to go down to investigate. First, I would gather up any kids in the house and put them into a bedroom (or safe room) with an adult if possible. Then I'd arm myself with an incidental weapon. I'd go downstairs and switch on all the lights to illuminate the area, so I can see what's ahead of me. I'd cautiously enter each room.

If I encountered an intruder, I would try not to put myself between him and any potential exit route from the house. I would say: 'The police have been called and are on their way. I'm giving you the chance to get out of the house.' Nine times out of ten, they'll leave. If they don't, you've got a problem: it probably means they're prepared to be aggressive toward you and your family, and you have to act pre-emptively. For me, this is when the situation starts to require violent action. If the intruder's not willing to leave, you have to put him down.

FIGHTING BACK

I would always advise evasive manoeuvres and de-escalation of potentially violent situations where possible. If an intruder is in your house to steal your property, let them have it. Even if it's an expensive item of jewellery, or one of great sentimental value, it isn't worth risking your life for. That's what you're doing if you fight back.

Sometimes, though, you're in a corner. Your family's safety might be at risk. Somebody might be in your house not to rob you but to do you harm, and you have no safe place to go. In such instances, I refer you to the chapter on how to fight. But you also need to know what the law says about confronting intruders in your own house. The good news is: the law's on your side. It is very uncommon for a householder to be prosecuted on account of using force against an intruder. In a nutshell:

- Wherever possible, you should call the police.
- You may use reasonable force to protect yourself and others, or to prevent crime.
- The more extreme the circumstances, the more force you may reasonably use.
- You do not have to wait to be attacked before using force.

Even if you accidentally kill an intruder, you are not at fault provided you have used reasonable force. This doesn't mean you can administer limitless violence, however. You cannot use 'disproportionate' force. For example, if you knocked an intruder unconscious, then continued to lay into them, you would be at fault. Similarly, if you hunted down an intruder and acted out of revenge, or set a trap for an intruder whom you knew was coming, rather than calling the police.

At night, again I would always recommend having something solid, like a baseball bat, near to hand. Hopefully you'll never have to use it, but it could save your life. (If you're going to keep a baseball bat in your safe room, or in any other location, for use as a weapon, keep a baseball ball with it. That way you can't be accused of carrying a dangerous weapon with intent to harm.)

Choke points

In military strategy, a choke point is a narrow channel through which an enemy force has to pass to get from one place to another. A choke point reduces a force's combat effectiveness by limiting its movement. That makes it a good defensive position for a smaller force.

Your house has choke points. Think staircases. If I had to defend my family against an intruder and I had no safe room, I would get my family on to the first floor and position myself at the top of the staircase. (I would even stand here if I *did* have a safe room, while my family made themselves secure.) At the top of the stairs, I would have the tactical advantage of height, and I would know that there was only one route the intruder could take to get to my loved ones. That one route means getting past me first. I would arm myself with my baseball bat, or whatever improvised weapon I could find, and I would defend that choke point to the death.

Tactical positioning

If you're in a safe room and an intruder is trying to gain access through an unblockaded door, your best position for counter-attacking is next to the door, by the opening. Grab an incidental weapon — the old baseball bat is good, but any solid, heavy bludgeon will do – and as soon as a head or any body part breaches that gap, hit it as hard as you can.

Don't position yourself in front of the door. If it comes flying in, it'll hit you and knock you back (as my wife found out when we were dating!)

CHRIS RYAN'S HOME SECURITY DEBRIEF

- Think like a thief.
- The obvious entry points are the most common, so brace your doors and secure your windows.
- Avoid opening your door to unknown, unvetted, unexpected individuals.
- Don't try to outwit a thief with crafty hiding places. They've seen it all before. Get a safe you can bolt to the floor or wall.
- Consider a safe room and identify choke points.
- You can use reasonable force to defend yourself and your family against an intruder in your house.

6

CYBER SECURITY

When the terrorist cell I referred to in the opening pages of this book targeted my daughter, they identified her on account of her online presence. This was a sharp reminder to us as a family that, for all the benefits it brings, the internet is also a powerful tool for anyone who wants to do us harm. We're not only talking about people stealing our credit card numbers. What we do online can have a real and devastating effect on our safety in the real world.

Of course, the internet is also a hotbed of opportunistic crime. With so many tens of millions of transactions being carried out every day on the internet, a criminal doesn't need a very high hit rate to make it worth his or her while.

Just as in the real world, it's not possible to be completely secure online. In the wake of Edward Snowden's leaks about the US government's surveillance capabilities, the Kremlin started using typewriters rather than computers for sensitive documents. If the security services can hack the Kremlin, they can hack you. And if the security services can do it, so can entities whose intentions are more sinister.

But it is possible to make yourself *more* secure. There are some simple precautions you can take to keep you and your family safe online. You need to be on top of this stuff to stay safe in the modern world. You also need to understand that you can't simply use one security method and ignore all the others, any more than you would lock your front door when you're away, but keep all your windows open. Cyber criminals are extremely sophisticated – much more sophisticated than street criminals or burglars. And because the vast majority of their attacks are automated, you need to be quite clear that the internet that you use daily is under constant attack. At some point, you *are* going to draw fire. Think of each of the points in this chapter as the individual components of a suit of body armour. Individually, they won't necessarily protect you. Together, they form a strong defensive barrier.

DON'T BROADCAST YOUR LOCATION OR PERSONAL INFORMATION

In this chapter, I'm going to explain some of the technical threats to which we're exposed online, and what you can do to combat them. But the first thing I want you to remember is this: *you* are a defensive layer.

I've spoken a lot about situational awareness in the real world. It applies equally online. We are encouraged to share the minutiae of our lives, and lots of people – often the most vulnerable ones – do this without thinking. When it comes to personal safety, this can be a catastrophic mistake.

You'd never put a sign outside your house stating: 'Occupants not at home'. It would make you an obvious target for thieves.

Every time you check in on Facebook, or announce your location in any way on social media, that's exactly what you're doing. If you have 500 friends on Facebook, and each of them has a similar number, and your privacy settings are set so that friends of friends can see your updates, you're broadcasting your location to a quarter of a million people. Is that really what you want to do? Even if you're only broadcasting to 100 friends, do you really know each of those people well enough to trust them completely?

Similarly, do you really want to broadcast your place of work? All it takes is one phone call to check that's where you are on a Thursday afternoon, and a potential burglar can break into your house knowing you're safely at your desk.

Criminals harvest information from your social media sites in more subtle ways, too. Details such as your name, address and date of birth can be used for identity theft. Personal information such as your mother's maiden name or your favourite film can be used to guess the security questions for your online accounts.

This is all private information and you should keep it private. Lots of people aren't aware that personal information they've shared with a social network is being broadcast by it. If you must share potentially sensitive information on social networks, take time to check your privacy settings very carefully – not all networks default to the most secure options.

Think carefully about any information you put in 'out of office' email replies. Stating that you're out of the country until a particular date is not necessarily information that you want to be broadcast.

Most phones have geo-location capabilities that automatically give information to certain apps about your location. Most of the time this is not necessary, and you can deny access to this information on an app by app basis. I always do this.

Sometimes, important information about ourselves ends up online without us really knowing about it. A good example of this is house-sale websites. An agent comes round, takes photographs of the interior of your house and puts it up online for the whole world to see. It's a gift to thieves: they can see the layout of your house (most of these websites even include flat plans of your property), they can see the strength of your door and window security, and crucially they can see if you have anything worth stealing. They can even detect personal information. I have, before now, looked at photographs of houses for sale in Hereford and been able to identify a couple belonging to members of the SAS, simply by seeing the military memorabilia hanging on their walls.

> When people think of cyber security, they normally imagine faceless hackers and financial scams. In fact, the reality can be personal and violent.
>
> At 2.30 a.m. on 3 October 2016, criminals dressed as police officers entered a luxury hotel complex on Rue Tronchet in Paris. The concierge was fooled by their uniform and let them through. Armed, they entered the apartment of the American reality TV star Kim Kardashian. They put a gun to her head and wrapped duct tape round her mouth. They tied her up, put her in the bath and locked the bathroom. They then stole £9 million worth of jewellery.

In my opinion, Kim Kardashian was lucky to be alive. In a situation like that, with live firearms, nervous criminals and large sums of money involved, anything could happen.

However, the situation could also have been prevented. In the days leading up to the robbery, Kardashian had posted pictures of her jewellery on Instagram. In the hours before, as she was getting dressed for a fashion event, she posted pictures of herself in her hotel room. Even if it wasn't common knowledge that this was where she normally stayed when in Paris, the interior of the hotel could be identified by similar publicity shots freely available on the internet. And she had posted a shot of herself in the hotel room moments before the robbery happened.

In short: the thieves knew where she was and they knew she had something worth stealing. She had unwittingly given them all the information they needed.

SECURE METHODS OF COMMUNICATION

Secure communications are crucial in the military. During the Bravo Two Zero mission, a lack of secure comms was a big problem when we initially deployed into Iraq. We had an encrypted radio to send messages back to base, but it was useless to us, because we'd been given the wrong frequencies. Our back-up option was a satellite communication device, but this was not encrypted. We knew that, if we used it, it would give off a big splash that could enable enemy forces to pinpoint our location. We had to risk it, and I don't know if anyone was listening in. But by that time, our location had been blown by other means anyway.

It's not only soldiers who should be aware of the potential weaknesses in their communications. I was recently talking to somebody very high up at MI6. We agreed to keep in touch, but he had a word of warning for me: on no account was I to text or email him. Any correspondence we had was to take place using the WhatsApp messaging app. Why? Because texts and emails can easily be hacked. WhatsApp, on the other hand, employs 'end-to-end encryption'. This is a way of encoding information so that the only people who can read the messages are the sender and the receiver. Not even the service provider can decrypt the message.

WhatsApp is not the only messaging service that provides this encryption, and it's controversial. Be in no doubt that this is how terrorists and other criminals communicate with each other. However, if it's good enough for MI6, it's good enough for me. I always try to use services with end-to-end encryption when I'm communicating with people online.

PASSWORD SECURITY

Your online passwords are like the locks on your house. If they're weak, you're asking to be broken into. If somebody breaks into your online accounts, the harm they can do you is immense. I'm not just talking about financial harm. Think of the information somebody could glean if they had access to your email. Again, they might learn when you are planning to be away from home, or that you've had delivery of some expensive TV equipment. If you're a lone female, they might be able to track your movements. They might find out where your kids go to school.

For these reasons, password security should be second nature to all of us. In my opinion, it's the single most important component to our online safety. Yet so many people have weak, insecure passwords. A five-letter password can be hacked, using software freely available on the internet, in a matter of minutes. If we increase that password to ten letters, it would take years to hack by brute force.

However, length isn't the only factor that makes a password hard to hack. It should also:

- Contain a mixture of lower-case letters, capital letters, numbers and symbols. This massively increases the number of possible options for each element of the password, which makes the password much more difficult to guess.
- Not contain dictionary words or well-known phrases. Password-hacking software prioritises strings of letters that form existing words.
- Not contain personal information about yourself.

There are some other password rules you need to follow:

- Use a different password for each login. I guarantee that if someone gets your password for one account, they'll try it on lots of other accounts.
- Change your passwords regularly – every six months or so.
- Never send a password to somebody in an email.
- Don't type it into a computer that doesn't belong to you or that you don't trust (see the section below on key-loggers).

A good password looks like this: 6%k=5eaAYVu (although please don't use this one). If we're following the rules above, we'll have a different one for every account. Obviously, none of us are going to remember a password like that. So I'd advise using a piece of software called a password manager. These are secure vaults on your computer that create super-secure passwords, encrypt them securely (the good ones use end-to-end encryption) and remember them for you, which is crucial, because good passwords are very obscure and purposefully unmemorable. You only need to know one master password. The machine does the rest.

TWO-FACTOR AUTHENTICATION

If you follow the advice above, it will be extremely difficult for a hacker to *guess* or *hack* your password. However, people can find your passwords by other means. Maybe the service you're trying to access has been hacked and its user passwords stolen *en masse*. Maybe you've written your password down somewhere and it's been stolen. Maybe someone has simply looked over your shoulder as you've typed it in.

Two-factor authentication is a countermeasure to these scenarios. It's a way of getting a user to prove that they are who they say they are, which in turn makes you more resilient to attack. If you bank online, you probably already use it when you're asked to type in a numerical code generated by an app or a dedicated key pad. You may not be aware that various other services – Google, Twitter, Facebook – offer something similar. Google, for example, provides a service whereby each time you try to log in, they will send a numerical code to your phone. If you can't enter this, you're locked out.

VPN

Every communication we make over the internet can potentially be read by a third party. Every website we visit can be logged. Our online behaviour can be examined. Governments do it. Security agencies do it. Commercial companies do it.

And criminals do it. All the time.

Cyber criminals have the capability to scan the internet looking for vulnerable computers and insecure communications.

A VPN is a virtual private network. They are fairly easy to set up on your computer, and they allow you to encrypt your connection to the internet and to remain anonymous online. As with WhatsApp and other encrypted messaging services, VPNs are often used by people flouting the law, but they are an essential tool for any law-abiding internet user wishing to minimise the risk of being 'overheard' while they're online.

Do your research. Not all VPNs are the same. Some are free, some have a small charge. The free ones tend to be less secure.

HTTPS

Get on to the internet and go to a website. In the browser's address bar, you'll probably see that the web address starts either with *http://* or with *https://*.

If it starts with the former, you need to know that everything you view on that website, every click you make and every search term you enter, can be viewed by a third party hacking the connection between you and the website.

If it starts with *https://*, a limited amount of information is still available, such as the domain of the site you are accessing, but the clicks and searches aren't.

I would be extremely wary of any website that doesn't use the *https* protocol. I certainly wouldn't enter any credit card or personal details on to an *http* site.

(Clue: the extra 's' stands for 'secure'.)

OTHER INTERNET SECURITY ESSENTIALS

As well as the above, you should always:

- Use antivirus software and keep it up to date. As well as protecting you from computer viruses, it will probably include a firewall that protects your computer from external attack.
- Keep your operating system and applications such as internet browsers constantly up to date. These updates almost always include security fixes and patches for known vulnerabilities.
- Stay clear of public wi-fi, especially for banking or other secure transactions. It's incredibly insecure.

PHISHING

If a random person came up to you on the street and asked for your bank details or your address, you wouldn't give it to them. The same holds true online. Phishing is when cyber criminals try to get you to give up your personal details willingly, if unwittingly. Some phishing attempts are very crude and obvious, others are quite sophisticated.

If you receive an email, a text or a phone call that purports to be from a real company and asking you to provide sensitive information, or to click on a link, be very wary. Contact the company first, by finding their official details independently, to check it's not bogus.

There are certain indicators that an email might be a phishing attempt:

- The subject line has odd spellings. This is done to fool your spam filter.
- 'Dear . . .' followed by your email address. If the person sending the email seems to know your address but not your name, be suspicious.
- You're being cajoled to act quickly for urgent reasons: your bank account has been hacked, or you're entitled to a reward if you act quickly.

Don't get complacent because you think you can spot phishing attacks a mile off. A very switched-on friend of mine had to get an ESTA permit to enter the United States. She was fooled by a bogus site, which took her money, but didn't supply the permit. (There are also sites that charge an extra fee, which you don't need to pay if you go to the official site, but they do also supply the ESTA.) When she had to apply for a second ESTA for her family, she was on the lookout for the scam, but got tricked again by a different site. Phishing attempts can be difficult to identify.

MALWARE

Malware is 'malevolent' software that gets downloaded on to your computer. Bugs, bots, spyware, Trojan horses, viruses – they can compromise your computer, steal data and even take control of your machine. You don't necessarily need to know all the types of malware. You just need to understand how to prevent it.

Your first line of defence against malware is the use of anti-virus software and ensuring you keep your operating system and other software up to date, as above. (You can download antivirus software, and a little independent research will soon tell you which is the best for your purposes.) But you must also be vigilant when it comes to downloading files from the internet, or opening email attachments from sources you don't trust. These are both common ways of infecting a person's computer with malware. Never open an attachment if you don't know who it's from.

If your computer starts running slowly or acting strangely, you need to make a priority of running some antivirus software on it. There's a chance that a piece of malware might be logging your keystrokes, in which case your personal information is no longer secure, or even that the webcam or microphone on your laptop could have been taken over, and you're being spied on. (For this reason, it's a good idea to have a piece of masking tape stuck over your webcam when it's not in use.)

CHRIS RYAN'S CYBER SECURITY DEBRIEF

- If you broadcast personal details or any information about your whereabouts on social media, your safety is immediately compromised.
- Passwords need to be long, obscure and unique.
- Passwords aren't foolproof. Use two-factor authentication whenever it's available.
- Virtual private networks keep you safe from prying eyes.
- Be suspicious about attachments, links and downloads. Remember: *you* are a defensive layer when it comes to cyber security.

7

HOW TO AVOID BEING SCAMMED

Scams are big business. In the UK alone we lose billions of pounds to scammers every year. Identity theft causes untold harm and distress.

But it's not only our financial security that is at risk from scammers. Our personal safety is under threat, too. To illustrate this, I want to tell you the story of a guy called Mike (not his real name), who received a stock email from a Nigerian scammer to tell him he could claim more than £3 million from a dead Nigerian family with the same surname. Mike told them to forget it and they went quiet for a while. Some months later, however, he received another email saying they needed to deposit a cheque for £100,000 into Mike's bank account, which he should then return to them to show that he was trustworthy. Still Mike declined. The next thing he knew, he had received a call from the scammers at his own home. The call didn't come from Nigeria, but from his home town. Mike got the police involved and thankfully he and his family remained safe. But there have been instances of people falling for similar scams, travelling to Nigeria and being kidnapped or even murdered. Some victims have committed suicide.

Or take the young British woman who was the victim of a 'crash for cash' scam. Polish gang members planned to crash their vehicle into a Transit van, in order to claim personal injury compensation. They got it wrong and hit the young woman's car. She was stranded in the fast lane of the motorway and was hit by another vehicle. She died.

The point is this: scammers are not the lovable rogues we see on *Hustle* or in Ealing comedies. They're not harmless spivs. They're dangerous criminals. Sometimes they're opportunistic and working alone. Sometimes they're backed by the machinery of organised crime. If you engage with them, you're engaging with potentially violent individuals with criminal tendencies, who display a complete lack of empathy and whose profession requires them to put their own needs above the safety of their victims.

Some scams are crude and rudimentary. Others are massively subtle and complex. Your first line of defence against them is to be aware that they exist and that you *are* a potential target. Don't fool yourself that it's only the naive and ignorant who get scammed. It isn't. It has happened to me, and recently. I was in the States, needing to fill my car up at a gas station. There was a card reader on the front of the petrol pump. I knew that there was a scam whereby the fronts of these card readers are replaced with false ones that scan your card and read your PIN number. You can identify real ones because they have a special hologram sticker. I failed to check for the sticker. A week later, it became clear that somebody was living the high life in Orlando with my card details. I kind of blame myself: I let my focus slip, failed to look for the hologram, forgot that I was a potential target, and I paid the price. I also failed to adhere to one of my personal rules, which is that I always try to stop for fuel in less dodgy, less run-down parts of town, where you're less likely to be targeted, scammed or attacked.

In this chapter, I'm going to explain some of the most common scams out there, so you'll recognise them if you encounter them. First, however, I'm going to explain one of the essential skills of an undercover operative, which I believe will help you stay safe from many scammers. It is the art of detecting whether somebody is lying to you.

HOW TO TELL WHEN SOMEONE IS LYING

SAS men are taught to lie. Often their lives depend on it. If you're working undercover, you need a cover story. For that cover story to be convincing, it must be detailed. If I were to ask you where you went to school, you'd be able to reply instantly, without hesitation. If you were pretending to be someone else, and you hadn't thought about the answer to this question, you'd hesitate. In the secret world, that moment of hesitation means you're blown. So SAS men rehearse their lies. They expand them, and drill deep into the details. The entire backstory of their new identity becomes second nature to them.

SAS men are also taught *not* to lie. If you're captured, you give your name, rank and number. Nothing else. As soon as you start inventing a cover story on the spot and entering into a dialogue with an interrogator, chances are that they'll keep revisiting things you've said as they try to pick holes in it. They'll catch you out eventually.

When we do tell a lie, we try to make it as close to the truth as possible. Obviously, if you're from Newcastle, there's no point saying you're from Liverpool. But when you're making up a backstory, you would say you came from an area of Newcastle that you know well, otherwise you'll expose yourself as a liar by not knowing simple facts about the area. You should be similarly careful about making up a profession you know nothing about. There's no point saying you're a mechanic if you're not: all an enemy has to do is present you with a broken Land Rover and tell you to fix it. If you can't, you're blown.

What we need to take away from this is that somebody who is trying to scam you may have a very good cover story, which they have worked on in minute detail, and which will probably be close enough to the truth that you'll find it hard to catch them out by asking them questions. But it is possible, with a little skill, to establish when someone's lying.

Lie-detecting is, of course, an imprecise art. Polygraph tests can be fooled, and some people are simply better at lying than others. Moreover, although there are certain physical 'clues' that someone might be lying to you, you can't rely on those alone. There's no point me telling you that scratching your nose is a sign of lying, if you're about to interview someone with hay fever!

Before you can make a judgement about a person's truthfulness or lack of it, you need to observe them first. It's the old jungle technique again, which we've been applying on the street, in our car and in our home. We need a heightened level of awareness, and an acute sense of what is *normal*. Only then can we make a judgement as to whether something *isn't* normal.

If I was trying to work out if a target was lying to me, I'd do my research first. I'd find out a bit about him or her. Inconsequential, innocent stuff that they wouldn't bother lying about. Do they have any brothers or sisters? Where do they work? I'd also try to find out something a bit less innocent, that they *would* want to lie about. Have they ever been in trouble with the police? Do they have a criminal record?

When we came face to face, I would first do everything I could to put them at their ease. I'd make them comfortable. I'd offer them a drink. We'd shoot the shit. I'd observe their behaviour when they were completely relaxed. This would give me a baseline from which to work: a point of comparison.

I'd then start asking the questions that my target has no reason to lie about. As I say, I'm likely to have done my research, but if you're doing this in a non-military scenario, this may not be possible. Let's say a salesman has come round to your house to talk about selling you some new windows. Keep it innocent. Ask him where he's going on holiday. Is he married? Does he have any kids?

I'd observe how they respond to these questions. What are their facial expressions? Do they seem nervous? Do they look away before answering? I'll make a mental note of any small gestures or idiosyncrasies. I now know that I can discount these as indicators that the subject is lying. If they change when I continue questioning them, it's a red flag.

I'd then change my questioning slightly. I'd start introducing questions to which I know the answer, but which they might lie about. In our non-military scenario, I might have done some research about our salesman's company and discovered some negative feedback. I'd watch him carefully as he denies it, noting any gestures or facial tics that he displays as he's lying.

I now know something about my target's behaviour. I've established what he looks like when he's telling the truth, and what he looks like when he's lying. Only then will I start asking him the questions in which I'm really interested.

The more you do this, the more you become adept at identifying untruthful behaviour. What follows is a list of possible indicators. None of them is a smoking gun by itself, and they are all dependent on the 'normal' behaviour of your target (someone might answer quickly, or stutter, or stare by default, in which case these indicators are of no use). But if you notice groups of these behaviours, you might be on to something.

The quick answer

People normally pause before answering a question. If they don't, and they seem to answer that little bit too quickly, it's a sign that they're giving you a pre-prepared response. I'd be suspicious of that. However, I'd also be suspicious of . . .

Stuttering

Even the best liars sometimes have a moment of anxiety before delivering a lie. But they quickly recover, and you can miss it if you're not looking for it.

The stare

It's a bit of a myth that people avoid your gaze when they're lying to you. In fact, they're more likely to maintain eye contact, in an effort to convince you that they're telling the truth.

The legs

Liars are adept at keeping control of their facial movements. They tend to be less conscious of their legs and feet. If a person starts twitching their feet or generally altering the movement of the lower part of their body when before it was still, it can be a sign that they're lying. I'd also look out for a particular stance where the target's torso is facing me, but his feet are directed toward the exit. This is often an indicator of lying.

Head-shaking

This can be a very subtle movement, but you can sometimes detect a faint shaking of the head when a target is lying.

Overreacting

If you confront somebody about a potential lie and their reaction is an over-the-top denial, it often means they really are lying.

Avoiding the answer

If your target answers a question with another question, or seems to be avoiding the question in any other way, he's probably lying.

However, just because they're *not* avoiding the question, it doesn't mean they're telling the truth. A good technique is to ask the same question in two or three different ways. If you find that your target uses the same form of words for each reply, it's an indication that they're working from a pre-planned script. Ask yourself why.

SOME COMMON SCAMS TO LOOK OUT FOR

Ponzi schemes and pyramid selling

These are both investment schemes that seem to offer massive returns. In a Ponzi scheme, the scheme manager doesn't invest the money, but keeps recruiting new investors and using their money to pay existing ones. As soon as the number of investors stops increasing, and it eventually will, the scheme collapses. (If you want to know more about Ponzi schemes, I'd recommend watching the Robert de Niro movie *The Wizard of Lies*, about Bernie Madoff, who ran the most famous Ponzi scheme of recent years.)

In a pyramid scheme, the investors themselves have to recruit new investors, and share the proceeds with people higher up the pyramid.

Both these schemes are scams. If somebody offers you something that seems too good to be true, it *is* too good to be true. In general, this is good advice to protect you from financial scams of all types.

Vishing

In the previous chapter we spoke about 'phishing'. Vishing is the telephone version of this. Somebody calls you up and tries to persuade you to hand over your bank details or other personal information. At the very start of this book, I told you about the phone call I received from the Midlands anti-terrorist unit. I refused to continue the conversation until I had verified the caller's identity. I advise that you do this every time you speak to an unknown person on the telephone, especially if they are asking you for any kind of personal details. Vishing calls are made every second. Note that banks will never ask you for your passwords over the phone. If someone does that, they're a fraud.

Crash for cash

If one car drives into another, it is usually the driver behind who is considered to be at fault for not keeping the correct stopping distance. Crash for cash incidents occur when the driver in front stages an accident so that they can make insurance claims for damage to their vehicle and personal injury.

If you suspect that this has happened to you:

- Admit *no* liability for the accident.
- Use your phone to take pictures of the scene and vehicle damage.
- Photograph the occupants of the other car – scammers often say there were more people in the car, so that they can claim extra money for personal injury.
- Don't tell the other driver you suspect them of scamming you, but insist on calling the police – they will probably back off at this point.
- Check for other witnesses. However, you need to understand that scammers often plant bogus witnesses when they're planning one of these hits.

In the chapter on staying safe in your car, I recommended using dash cams. This is another scenario in which they can be helpful.

Nigerian 419 scams

These are scams that originated in Nigeria, but which now come from other parts of the world. Scammers claim that they need to transfer money out of their country and ask for your bank account details to make the transfer, in return for a cut. Alternatively, they will ask you to pay a fee to facilitate the transfer.

These scams mostly arrive by email, but they can arrive by phone, post, text or over social networking. They often seem comically obvious, but they are presented in that way for a very good reason: it ensures that only the most vulnerable people reply. And reply they do: these scams work often enough for the scammers to continue doing them. You should never give bank details or arrange to transfer money in any way for someone you don't know. Perhaps more importantly, if you are responsible for a vulnerable person, such as an elderly relative, you need to make very sure that they are not being drawn into a scam of this type.

It is very important never to engage with people involved in this sort of scam, even for a joke. It might seem like a laugh to wind them up, but remember that you are dealing with criminals. They will likely pounce on anyone who engages with them.

INDICATORS THAT YOU'RE BEING SCAMMED

Unsolicited contact

Scammers will often contact you out of the blue. Of course, this is sometimes true of *bona fide* companies, too. In either case, you should always verify the identity of an unknown person who contacts you.

Request to share personal info

If you can't verify who you're talking to, don't give them *any* information about yourself – and certainly no sensitive financial information.

Pressure for a quick response

If you're offered a deal, but are being pressured into making a quick decision, walk away. Genuine companies and salesmen will always give you space to think, and a cooling-off period. Never hand over your money under pressure.

You're asked to keep things quiet

Why should you? Red flag.

CHRIS RYAN'S ANTI-SCAMMING DEBRIEF

- Don't assume that you won't fall for a scam. They can be very sophisticated and hard to spot. Your first line of defence is to be aware that you are a target.

- To tell if someone is lying, first you must observe how they act when they're telling the truth.
- Learn some of the common indicators that a person might be lying.
- If someone contacts you out of the blue, let suspicion be your default setting.
- Never engage with scammers. Remember that they are criminals, and a potential threat to your safety and that of your family.

8

KEEPING CHILDREN AND THE ELDERLY SAFE

Sometimes, keeping ourselves safe isn't enough. Many of us are responsible for potentially vulnerable people who can be targets for different types of threat – namely children and the elderly. It's important that we're aware of these, and that we take steps to mitigate against them.

THE ELDERLY

The elderly, especially those who live alone, are often at risk.

Sometimes they are at risk from themselves. Sometimes they are at risk from criminals and scammers. This is because they exhibit certain characteristics that predators home in on. They often have lump sums of money. They are often isolated and alone. They are often frail. They are often not very confident with technology. They may suffer from cognitive illnesses such as dementia or Alzheimer's. These characteristics make them a target.

Much of the advice in the chapter on staying safe in your home applies to the elderly, and it is crucial that elderly people are made aware of all the various types of scam and how to respond to them. There are, however, a few other tips I would like to give you if you find yourself responsible for an ageing parent, family member or friend.

Make an assessment of their environment

Just as you should make an objective assessment of your own home for security (see pages 82–9), so you should assess the security of an elderly person's house. Where are its weak spots? Have you fortified all points of entry? Are all the security measures in place? If anything, we need to be even more rigorous about this when we are dealing with the dwelling of a potentially vulnerable person: a burglar is much more likely to risk the home of a person who can't easily fight back. An elderly person's home should be a stronghold.

You should also assess an elderly person's house for trip and slip hazards, and ensure that there is proper internal lighting so they can always see where they're going. Occupational therapists will often visit a house to make sure it is as safe as possible for an elderly relative.

Ensure they can be identified

I would always encourage an elderly person to have a card in their wallet or purse with their name, address, a list of any medication they are on, and an emergency number such as yours. If they get lost, disorientated or have a bad turn while they're out, the police will be able to identify them immediately. It's a small detail that substantially increases their safety.

Make use of HD wi-fi cameras

On page 91, I recommended the use of security cameras on the exterior of your house. If you're responsible for an elderly person, I would suggest considering cameras inside the house, too.

This may be a difficult subject for you to broach. Nobody wants their privacy to be invaded, and I certainly wouldn't suggest placing a camera in bathrooms or bedrooms. However, if the elderly person has an accident in one of the other rooms and collapses, a camera in that room will alert you. If they fail to leave their bedroom or bathroom in the morning, that's another alert.

If an elderly person understands that this a safety measure, they may agree to it. If not, you might suggest sensor monitoring. These are smart systems that detect changes in a person's usual patterns of movement, and alert a loved one if something out of the ordinary seems to be happening.

In terms of personal safety, wi-fi cameras really come into their own at the front door. Security cameras are a criminal's worst nightmare. Cameras make their presence at a crime scene a matter of record, and can even record what they say. If I was responsible for an elderly person, I would always ensure that there is a wi-fi camera at the front door, facing any callers. If an unknown person comes to the door, the elderly person can clearly state that the caller needs to speak on the camera to their son, daughter or whoever is their main carer. I guarantee that this will be a good line of defence against unscrupulous predators.

I would also have no hesitation in setting up a covert wi-fi camera in the room of a family member if they were staying in a care home. There have been horrific incidents of abuse of the elderly in a small minority of care homes. These occur because the abusers know that their victims may be too confused to be believed if they complain. Setting up a camera removes a predator's ability to act uncensored.

It's not foolproof, however. So I refer you to the SAS's double camera trick, as described on page 91. If a predator has disabled a visible camera, they won't be thinking to look for a second covert one. That's how you catch them.

GPS trackers

When an SAS team is on an operation, each member of the unit has a GPS tracker built into their radio pack. This means that when they're operating in a threatening environment, the command centre knows their precise location at all times.

We can use the same technology to keep our elderly loved ones safe. It can be very distressing when an elderly person leaves the house and can't be found, not to mention dangerous for them. There are a number of GPS tracking devices that enable you to locate them quickly if they wander. Some of these simply go into a pocket or on a key ring. Some come as bracelets and some are even built into shoes or insoles so they can't be forgotten. You can attach GPS trackers to vehicles for elderly people who are still driving.

Panic alarms

These are worn on the wrist or around the neck. If the wearer activates the alarm, a control centre calls their number. If they get no response, they call the next of kin. It's an effective way to help an elderly person who has had a fall or is in difficulty.

Guarding against scammers

Everything in the chapter on how to avoid being scammed holds true. However, you need to remember that elderly people are more at risk from the unscrupulous, and this risk can sometimes come from unexpected sources. I have an aunt who, unbeknown to her family, had been pressured into donating to more than a hundred different charities by hard-sell door-to-door and telephone sales people on a commission. When we realised what had happened, we got her to choose two or three of her favourites, then slash the rest. We then had her removed from cold-calling lists (register with the Telephone Preference Service to do this).

It's not only charities who target the elderly. There's a never-ending source of unscrupulous tradesmen lining up to tell worried pensioners that they need a new drive, or a new roof, or new doors or windows, when they really don't. It's important to encourage elderly people always to check with a family member before embarking on any type of work like that.

KEEPING CHILDREN SAFE

I take the view that the modern world is a very difficult place for a child to negotiate. I'm not here to give anybody any parenting advice, but I do want to give some tips with respect to what I believe to be the three greatest threats to the safety of children: cyberbullying, child abduction and online sexual predators.

Cyberbullying

I was bullied at school. It was the usual story: I was the small kid in the class and I got picked on by the bigger kids. They say that people are either prey or they're hunters. I was definitely the prey, and the hunt would happen outside the school gates, where a big crowd would gather to watch the fight. When it was over, I'd dust myself down and go home.

These were different times. One day I was in a fight. I lost and came home with a bleeding nose. My dad saw the state of me and asked me what had happened. I told him. 'Did you win?' he asked.

'No.'

'Then go round to this lad's house, knock on his door and tell him that you want another fight. If you don't, I'll drag you down there myself.'

I was horrified. But I did what I was told. I knocked on this boy's door, told him I wanted another fight, and got my arse kicked for a second time. I returned home in tears. 'Did you win?' my dad asked.

'No.'

'Then go back down and tell him you want *another* fight.'

I was shitting myself, but I did what he said. I returned to this lad's house three times, and eventually I learned the lesson that my father was trying to teach me. When someone punches you, it hurts. But if they keep on punching you, there comes a point where it doesn't hurt any more. That's what happened with me. It stopped hurting, I stopped being frightened, and I gave as good as I got. I ended up getting the better of the bully and he never touched me again.

Let me make myself clear: I'm not advocating this as a strategy, principally because the nature of bullying has changed. It doesn't stop at the playground gates. Modern bullying has gone virtual. Kids have to deal with their bullies needling them on social media from the moment they wake to the moment they go to sleep. There have been too many instances of young people hurting themselves and even committing suicide, because of the relentless bullying and negativity they receive online. It's psychological warfare, and while the physical attacks I had to endure did eventually stop hurting, these psychological ones don't. And whereas physical bullying often has physical signs – it's hard to hide a bleeding nose – cyberbullying often doesn't.

No human should be subjected to this, let alone kids. No young person should have to dread walking through the school gates every day. These are places of education, not battlegrounds. Our time there is short and not to be wasted on some idiot trying to make themselves look good by bullying.

To any young people reading, I say this: there is no shame in being bullied. It happened to me and it happens to lots of people. You can't sit on it and ride it out by yourself. You must always tell someone what is going on – your mum or dad, a brother or sister, or a teacher. There are systems in place to deal with this stuff, but they only work if you're open and honest with the people who care about you.

It is crucial that adults are hyper-alert to the signs of bullying. These include:

- Inexplicable injuries.
- Damaged belongings.
- Feigning illness and attempts to miss school.
- Coming home from school hungry, because they've skipped lunch to avoid their bullies.
- Nightmares and trouble sleeping.
- Poor school work.
- Becoming withdrawn, or demonstrating anxiety or aggression.
- Bed wetting.
- Reluctance to enter social situations and suddenly losing friends.
- Lack of self-esteem.
- Drug or alcohol abuse.
- Stealing money to give to a bully.
- Self-harming and suicidal talk.

If you notice any of these signs, speak to your child and to the school. There is lots of good advice on the NSPCC website.

Child abduction

This is a topic that nobody likes to think about. A child going missing is one of the most terrible outcomes imaginable. That's why we tend to be unprepared for it. But it happens. We shouldn't put our heads in the sand. We should prepare ourselves. I want to give you a few tips about how to do this.

When children go missing they are often found in the house. This happened to my daughter – I was ready to get the Regiment to seal off Hereford when we found her asleep under her bed. However, even though this is true, if you suspect your child has gone missing you must get on to the police immediately. The initial stages of a child abduction investigation are the most important. Police officers are trained to think in terms of the 'golden hour' – the first hour after the abduction, during which they can most effectively identify witnesses, secure crime scenes and track down suspects. They can put in cordons and flood the area with officers. After that hour, the process becomes much more difficult, and the police response less effective. And even *within* the golden hour, the risk to the abducted person increases with every second that passes. You literally have no time to lose.

Every parent should have an up-to-date picture of their child. Not a fun one, where they're pulling a funny face or wearing sunglasses on the beach. A standard, serious photograph, regularly updated, that can be used to identify the child. When a child goes missing, every second counts. You don't want to be wasting precious time finding a decent photograph to pass to the police, or giving them an old, blurred photo that helps no one. Have a good photo on your phone or in a safe place, so you can act quickly to get it distributed.

I would also make sure that I had a DNA sample of my child. This can be from a lock of hair or a finger-prick blood sample on a scrap of blotting paper. A DNA sample is not only for the identification of bodies, although that is one of their purposes. It can also be used to help *find* a missing person. If, for example, there was a report of a certain man abducting a young girl, having a DNA sample of the child would enable the police to swab the suspect's car. If they find traces, they know they've got their guy and have a higher chance of finding the child.

Just as there are GPS trackers available for the elderly, there are small GPS tracking tags that can be sewed into a child's clothes or rucksack. If I had a young child I would do this, so that I could tell where they were at all times. You might have trouble persuading a teenager that this was a good idea, but in this instance, I would make it a condition of them having their own phone that they keep its GPS tracker on at all times, so that you're in a position to locate them if the worst happens.

If you're on holiday, it's easy for your child to get separated from you. Always make sure they have a card with your name, phone number and the address of your hotel or wherever you're staying.

Online sexual predators

Forget any preconceptions you might have about sexual predators being dirty old men in macs. I was once doing a prison survey in the Category A wing at a UK prison. We were there to establish how the Regiment would respond in the event of a prison riot. As we were leaving, the wardens told us that the prison was about to get very noisy: it was time for the sex offenders to be let out of their cells for their break. Sure enough, there was an uproar, with the regular inmates screaming and shouting at the sex cases as they passed their cells.

But what struck me wasn't the noise. It was the sex offenders themselves. They were young, fit, good-looking guys, mostly in their twenties. Sure, there were a couple of scruffy old men, but they were a small minority.

Sex offenders aren't all of a type. You can't pick them out in the street. They're defined by their urges, not their appearance. And in the internet, they have a very powerful tool for grooming young people.

I have a friend in America who is in the police force. He specialises in catching sexual predators. We were talking about how easy it is for young people to be groomed online. 'Watch this,' he told me.

He took out his laptop and logged on to the website of a random school. He found a picture of a recent football match and identified one of the cheerleaders. Within a few minutes, he had found her name and her email address. He emailed her, pretending to be a new student at the school. The girl responded, asking if they'd met. 'We spoke briefly at the football game,' my friend told her, before telling her that he'd enjoyed the match and thought she looked great. The dialogue continued. My friend asked the girl if she fancied going to a party that Saturday. She agreed.

Within twenty minutes of my friend opening his laptop, he had snared this teenager into meeting someone she had never met.

My friend's demonstration was chilling, because it was all so easy. If he hadn't succeeded, he could simply have moved on to another cheerleader at another school. Eventually he would have entrapped someone.

On the chapter on cyber security, I emphasised how crucial it is not to place too much personal information online. This is especially important for children and young people. It is essential that young people understand these limits, and why they are important. They need to understand that sexual groomers can be male or female and that they can be any age. They must understand that 'stranger danger' applies as much to encounters on the internet as it does to encounters in real life.

It's unrealistic to imagine you can have complete control over and knowledge of your child's online activity. With this in mind, there are certain aspects about online behaviour that you should always discuss with your children:

- The internet is real life. You should behave online just as you behave in the real world. And you should understand that, like in the real world, there are good people online and there are bad people.
- They should always come to you if they encounter something or someone that makes them feel uncomfortable. Tell them you won't overreact or ban them from using their device – you just want to help them stay safe.
- Show them how they can stay safe on social networks by learning where the reporting functions are (so they can report inappropriate behaviour), how to block someone and how to keep information private. (If you don't know how to do this stuff yourself, look at the NSPCC Net Aware website.)
- Teach them to be wary of online 'friends' who aren't friends in real life, and of unknown people arranging to meet them or offering them something for nothing.
- Explain that *everything* they put on the internet has the potential to stick around for the rest of their lives. There have been instances of teenagers being placed on the sex offenders' register for sending inappropriate pictures to each other. Actions have consequences. It might seem like a bit of fun, but it can haunt you for the rest of your life.

Even if you do all this, you can't guarantee that your child will remain safe from online predators. It can be hard to tell if a child is being groomed. Indicators include:

- Secrecy, especially about their online activity.
- Older boyfriends or girlfriends.
- Meeting their friends in unusual places.
- Having new possessions that they couldn't otherwise afford and can't explain.
- Having access to alcohol and/or drugs.
- Exhibiting changes in behaviour, and especially exhibiting age-inappropriate sexual behaviour.

And of course, sexual grooming does not only happen online. Be aware that many sexual predators target the parents before they target the children. It is very common for abused children to know their abusers.

Coded SOS alerts

This is an old military trick, but one that can easily be adapted to a civilian situation. Set up an innocent-sounding distress code with your teenage child. The trick is that it mustn't *sound* like a distress code. 'I'm having a great time' or 'Can I stay an hour longer'. It just needs to be a form of words that you both understand. If your teenager texts or messages you this phrase, it means they are feeling uncomfortable in whatever social situation they find themselves. Trust their instincts. Your response should be to call back and state that there is a family emergency and you need to come and collect them. It's a good way of airlifting them out of a situation that they can't necessarily deal with themselves.

CHRIS RYAN'S ELDERLY AND YOUNG PERSONS' SAFETY DEBRIEF

- Make an environmental assessment of an elderly person's home.
- Make sure an elderly person can be identified if they get into trouble.
- Use technology: think HD cams and GPS systems.
- Cyberbullying is psychological warfare. Know the signs.
- Have an up-to-date photo and DNA sample of your child.
- Be aware of the signs of sexual grooming.
- Set up a coded SOS alert.

9

STAYING SAFE ON HOLIDAY

On 26 June 2015, at approximately 11.15 hours local time, a 23-year-old student by the name of Seifeddine Rezgui arrived at the Tunisian tourist resort of Port El Kantaoui on the Tunisian coast.

He did not look like a killer. He was dressed as a tourist and carried a beach umbrella. He made his way along the beach until he reached the vicinity of the Hotel Riu Imperial Marhaba. Here, he removed a Kalashnikov assault rifle from inside the beach umbrella. He opened fire on tourists lying on sun loungers on the beach.

There was understandable panic. Holidaymakers tried to flee. The gunman entered the hotel complex and continued his killing spree. He escaped back to the beach and into the local town. Approximately an hour after the atrocity began, he was shot dead by Tunisian security forces. An eye witness saw a grenade rolling from his hand as he died.

Thirty-eight people lost their lives. Thirty of them were British tourists.

The Tunisian beach bombings were an aberration. But they were not completely unpredictable. And although it is true that our responses to such a crime are limited, they are not non-existent. At the end of this chapter, I will give you some ideas of what they might be.

Here's the problem with holidays. We relax. Nothing wrong with that. But we also let our guard down. That's a big mistake.

It happens to almost everybody. We might be hyper-alert to threats in our everyday lives, but as soon as we go on holiday, we behave differently. Our situational awareness reduces when it should increase. Finding ourselves in an unfamiliar environment, we just go with it, rather than taking the time to make ourselves aware of our surroundings. We often drink more alcohol, and behave in ways that we wouldn't ordinarily behave at home. We dress and act like tourists, which means that rather than blend into our surroundings, we stick out. Our general behaviour on holiday makes us a target.

Of course, we all *want* to relax on holiday. I'm not here to tell you that you need to be so obsessed with your family's security that your holiday is ruined. But we *are* vulnerable when we put ourselves in different environments. So in this chapter, I also want to give you a few tips about how to reduce those vulnerabilities to keep you and your family safe on holiday.

FOREIGN OFFICE ADVICE

An SAS operative will always arm himself with as much local intel as possible before inserting into an unknown area. This information will come from a variety of sources, such as intelligence agents on the ground, GCHQ and MI6 communications intercepts, a detailed study of geographical features and expected weather patterns.

Not all of this, of course, is available to the civilian traveller. But plenty of advice *is* at our fingertips. The best source of that advice is the British government itself.

If you go to www.gov.uk/foreign-travel-advice, you will be able to access the UK government's official advice with respect to travel to individual countries. This advice is detailed and practical. I would always consult it before travelling to a different country. For example, as I write this, I am looking at the Foreign Office advice for France. Now, you might think that travelling somewhere as familiar as France doesn't require anything in the nature of extra personal security. I would disagree. The FO advice at the time of writing tells me that there's a national state of emergency and terrorist attacks are very likely. It directs me to a smartphone app that gives alerts for security incidents – natural, technological and terror-related risks. It warns of petrol shortages in certain areas, and much more. This is important information, and I want to have it before I travel.

At the time of the Tunisian beach shootings, the Foreign Office advice stated that there was a 'high risk of terrorism including kidnapping' and that 'attacks could be indiscriminate, including in places visited by foreigners'. It did not, however, advise against all travel to Tunisia.

It is clearly up to you what level of risk you are willing to take when you make the decision to journey abroad. Moreover, I do not know whether any of those affected by the shootings in Tunisia were aware of the travel advice before they decided to holiday there. What I can say is this: it is sometimes not enough to rely on one source of intelligence. If I was making a decision about whether or not to take my family on holiday to a part of the world where a specific threat is known to exist, the first thing I would do would be to look at a map. In the case of Tunisia, I would see that it shares two borders: one with Algeria, one with Libya. For me, this would ring two alarm bells.

Firstly, Algeria and Libya are not stable states. As I write this, travel is not advised along the Algerian/Tunisian border, as well as many other parts of Algeria. And the FO advises against all travel to Libya.

Secondly, the borders between these north African states are porous. They are not hard borders like we are used to in the UK. People can pass across them with ease. When I trekked across Iraq in the wake of the Bravo Two Zero mission, I was heading for the Syrian border. When I reached it, it was little more than a barbed wire fence, which I managed to cross even in my starving, dehydrated, hallucinating state.

It is a day's drive from the coastal holiday resorts of Tunisia to the badlands of Libya, where extremist groups are rife. I can guarantee that there are countless thousands of unregistered, unregulated firearms crossing those borders every year. In the UK, it's pretty tough (though by no means impossible) to acquire a firearm and go on the rampage in Margate. In north Africa, it really isn't. You can buy an AK-47 and a box of 7.62s at an Algerian souk one day, and be firing them at a beach full of tourists in Tunisia the next.

In short, I want you to look beyond the holiday brochures, the golden sands and the tempting swimming pools. If a tour operator tells you that travel to a particular region is perfectly safe, be like an SF operative and gather information about this important matter from more than one source. Check the Foreign Office advice, check the maps, check the history of violent activity in the surrounding area. Do your homework. Only then are you fully equipped to make the decision whether to travel to that part of the world or not.

Finally, be aware that many places we think of as holiday destinations can be dangerous if you stray into the wrong area, or come up against the wrong people. Take the USA, for example. It might be the land of Disney World, but let's not forget the two young British tourists who'd been out drinking in Florida and had mistakenly walked into a dangerous area, where a sixteen-year-old kid held them up at gunpoint and shot them through the heart when they said they had no money. As a civilian in America I've witnessed two armed robberies, and even a road-rage incident where two drivers argued over a parking spot and shot one another. It's very easy to become complacent in the States, as it is in Mexico, Cape Town, Jamaica, India, Thailand, Tunisia, Egypt, Indonesia, Turkey — all these holiday destinations, and many more, have their dangerous sides. You need to be aware of them if you want to keep yourself and your family safe.

FAMILIARISATION

When you arrive at a new holiday location, the temptation is to hit the beach the moment you get there. This is a mistake. Before you do anything else, you need to familiarise yourself with your surroundings. Find all the entrances to your hotel complex or other accommodation. Think: if there was an emergency, would you have an immediate exit strategy for you and your family? Take a walk around the surrounding area. Look for landmarks that you can recognise if you need to return to your hotel. Examine a map. Ask yourself: if there was a terror incident, or a fire, or any kind of emergency, would I know how to get myself to safety, or would I be running blindly through the streets?

Your aim in doing all this is not only to arm yourself with the requisite knowledge in case you need to respond to an emergency situation. It is also to stop you *looking* lost and confused. You'll remember from the chapter on staying safe in the street that an air of confidence is a powerful tool, if you don't want to present yourself as a target. This is equally true abroad as it is at home.

You need to be aware that dodgy areas and safe areas often butt up against each other. It can be very easy to wander from one to the other without knowing it. I would always research my destination before leaving home. When I'm there, I'd ask someone familiar with the locality if there are any areas I should avoid.

Arm yourself with certain pieces of information: the address and number of the nearest British embassy, high commission or consulate, the address and number of your hotel, and the local police numbers. Be aware that in some parts of the world, such as the US, there are a number of different police departments. Make sure you have the numbers for each. Plug these numbers into your phone and take them with you wherever you go. If there's an emergency situation, make the call – don't rely on someone else to do it.

Compile a list of safe places to go if you get into trouble. Police stations might be on this list, but be aware that in certain countries, the police may not provide a safe haven for a traveller in trouble. There are plenty of corrupt police forces in the world. Instead, you might head for a big, reputable hotel (but not dodgy, run-down ones), to a church or monastery, or to the airport. You can only know where safe havens are if you do your research first.

A good source of information is your hotel receptionist or concierge. They will know which areas are safe and which should be avoided. Don't ignore their advice, as my brother once did in the Dominican Republic. He was staying in an all-inclusive hotel complex. The staff advised him not to leave, because there was a lot of crime in the surrounding areas. My brother got bored of the complex and ignored their advice. He went to a bar a hundred yards up the road, where somebody attempted to rob him at knifepoint. (My brother's quite handy with his fists, so he punched the thug as soon as he saw the knife, which gave him enough time to leg it back to the complex.)

BLENDING IN

We've already spoken about the importance of choosing clothes that help you blend in to your surroundings. This is just as important when you're abroad. Unfortunately, most of us go in the opposite direction, dusting off that tropical shirt that we haven't worn since our last holiday, or walking the streets with an expensive camera round our neck. It's so important that you don't do this. Tourists are actively targeted by criminals in *every* holiday destination in the world. There's no exception. Tourists are generally carrying decent quantities of cash and they have lower levels of situational awareness. If you *look* like a tourist, you *are* a target. So: look around. What are the locals wearing? Can you emulate them? If you can, you should.

During my time in the SAS, there were tensions on the Zimbabwe–Botswana border. B Squadron were tasked with investigating the options for a covert insertion into Botswanan territory. Our plan was to take a commercial flight into Zimbabwe, then head west cross-country to infiltrate the Botswanan border.

We did this by utilising two important facts that I hope you will have taken away from this chapter. We knew that in order to get into Zimbabwe without ringing any alarm bells, we needed to disguise ourselves. A squadron-sized group of burly male 'tourists' would have appeared unusual. We needed to blend in, so at the airport we presented ourselves as rugby players on our way to a tournament. That got us into Zimbabwe with barely a question asked.

From that point on it was easy. The border between Zimbabwe and Botswana is porous, as so many African borders are. We were able to enter the country covertly. An entire SAS squadron was in situ without any of the local authorities realising we were there.

ATMOSPHERICS

When soldiers operate in potentially threatening urban environments, they learn to become extremely sensitive to the 'atmospherics' of the place — it means the mood, or vibe, that they encounter. You can patrol down a street one day and the atmospherics will be relaxed and unthreatening: kids playing, smiles from the locals. The following day they can change completely: no kids, and stares from the locals. Atmospherics inform a soldier's sense of his or her personal security just as much as more concrete intelligence. They learn not to ignore it.

We need to do the same in unfamiliar environments, especially when we're abroad and in parts of the world where sections of the local community may be resistant to our presence. If the locals appear unfriendly, or it's unusually quiet, or you simply feel uncomfortable in a particular part of town, go with your gut. Get out of there and don't return.

UNDERSTANDING LOCAL LAWS

I spend a lot of time in America, where people are allowed to carry firearms. In certain states, it is illegal to stand at a bar while you're carrying. So, if I see empty seats at the bar and a group of guys congregating at a high-top table nearby, I can be pretty sure they are armed.

In Thailand, it's illegal to criticise the royal family. People have been punished for 'liking' an insulting post on Facebook.

Wherever you go, you need to be sensitive to local customs and laws. It will help you blend in, and it will stop you getting into trouble. Do your research before you travel.

CARRYING MONEY AND VALUABLES

A bulging wallet in your back pocket is a magnet for a thief: you're telling them where your money is, and that there's a lot of it. Bum bags are a bit safer, but they're still an obvious target.

The safest place to carry money is the hardest to pickpocket. This is the breast pocket of a shirt, with a buttoned flap over it. Put a pullover on and it's impossible to pickpocket surreptitiously. Again, make sure there's no bulge. Just carry a small amount of cash and a card.

Don't wear a high-quality watch on holiday. Get a cheap one that will do the job. The same goes for expensive jewellery. If you're wearing either of these, you're advertising that you've got money. Thieves are switched on. They'll know the value of a Rolex or a Cartier. If it's particularly valuable, they'll more than pick your pocket – they'll cut your throat for it.

VEHICLE SAFETY

You are substantially more likely to die on the road in low- or middle-income countries than you are in the UK. Many of these countries are those that attract tourism. All the vehicle safety advice earlier in this book applies, but there are certain extra elements that we need to consider.

In general, in poorer parts of the world, I would avoid travelling by car after dark. This is when most accidents and crime occur.

When you're abroad, you'll probably find yourself using either taxis or hire cars. They each bring with them certain risks.

Taxis

Most people would never get into a vehicle with a stranger. Yet we do exactly this when we take a taxi. In certain parts of the world, that's fine. I'd feel completely comfortable about my family members taking a registered black cab in London. In other parts of the world, taxis can be high-risk. I would always want my family members to take the following precautions:

- Always get your hotel to pre-book a taxi to meet you at the airport or train station. These places are a magnet for unofficial cab drivers, who are far more likely to try to scam you or, worse, threaten your personal safety.
- If this isn't possible, always take taxis from official taxi stands.
- Check your taxi driver's ID and credentials before getting into his vehicle. There should be photo ID openly on display, the vehicle should have a radio and there should be a meter. If there are none of these, don't get in – no matter how much this might inconvenience you.
- Agree a price (an approximate one at least) and a route before you start. If you seem to be deviating from the route, make a fuss. Get out at a red light if you need to.
- If you're travelling alone, always position yourself in the back seat, behind the driver. It makes you less accessible to him if he has bad intentions. Certainly, never sit in the front seat where you are close at hand.
- Maintain the same level of vehicle security that you would at home. Keep your window shut, your door locked and your seatbelt on.

Hire cars

If you're driving in an unfamiliar country, all the usual safety advice applies. Additionally, you must make yourself aware of the rules of the road in whichever country you're driving. Don't assume that they're the same as in the UK, because they're not. In France, for example, if somebody flashes their headlamps at you, it can mean that they expect you to get out of their way. In the UK, it means they're giving way to you.

However, you need to be extra vigilant if you're in a hire car. They are specifically targeted by thieves and carjackers. In certain parts of the world, criminals position themselves close to the hire-car exit ramps at airports, knowing that these vehicles are likely to contain tired, disoriented tourists with plenty of ready currency, valuable documents for resale, and luggage.

Your first line of defence against this type of behaviour is, as always, a heightened level of awareness. Read the pages in this book on carjacking, and always drive on if you're flashed by another vehicle or even driven into. However, I would also always ensure that there is no indication that my car *is* a hire car by removing any hire-car company stickers from the windscreens. (In the US, rental car number plates used to be common. This is no longer the case, because they were a beacon for criminals.)

HOTEL SAFETY

For a criminal, a hotel is like a sweet shop. There are hundreds of temporary residents, many of whom are storing money, documents and expensive electrical equipment in their rooms, most of whom are less aware of their surroundings. Thieves can walk in and out of busy hotels without being challenged or even noticed. And while security systems are in place in most hotels, they are easily bypassed if the guests or hotel staff let their vigilance drop for a moment.

When undercover operatives are working abroad, hotels are often a fact of life. There are certain precautions I would always take, whether I'm on operations or not. I want these to become second nature to you when you're staying in a hotel.

Before you book

Try to stay in hotels that have electronic key cards rather than old-fashioned key locks. The electronic codes get changed every time there's a new guest. If a criminal gets a copy of a room key, which is easily done, they have access to the room until the lock is changed.

Many hotels require you to use your key card in the lift to get access to the guest floors. This is a good security measure.

When you check in

It's important to keep your personal details as private as possible from unscrupulous people who might overhear you as you check in. If somebody knows your full name and room number, your security is compromised, because it's then easy for people to pretend to be you and gain access to your room.

If you've pre-booked, always ask for a room change at the desk. If somebody is targeting you, they may have got hold of the hotel guest list. This way, they won't be able to match up your personal details to your room.

You may have noticed that in most hotels, the receptionist will write your room number on a slip of paper rather than saying it out loud. This is a security measure – it means anybody listening can't overhear your number. If the receptionist *does* say it out loud, ask for a room change.

Don't give your first name when checking in – just 'Mr' or 'Mrs' and your initial. Hotel guest lists are not secure, and this is one way of limiting the amount of personal information you give up. If you are a lone female, always say that you are a 'Mrs'. This will make anybody listening in suspect that you're not travelling alone.

Never accept a room on the ground floor. These are by far the easiest to break into. The safest rooms are generally between the second and the sixth floor – any higher than that and you're probably out of reach of fire-engine ladders.

Always ask for two key cards, for reasons that will become clear below.

In your room

If you have a mobile phone, call the hotel reception once you get to your room and ask to speak to yourself. If the receptionist announces your room number, you must immediately speak to the hotel management to make sure it doesn't happen again. Your room number is private, and a matter of personal security.

Put any valuables – including documents – in the room safe. If there isn't one, or you're not convinced that it's very secure, use the main hotel safe. Always get written confirmation of what you've stored in there.

If a hotel employee knocks on your door, *always* phone down to reception to verify their identity. It's a common tactic for intruders to pose as employees.

When you arrive in your room, you have two immediate priorities. The first is to check your exit routes. Try to imagine the last time you stayed in a hotel. Now, be honest with yourself: if you'd become aware that there was a shooting on the ground floor and the gunmen had knocked the electricity out, or if there was a fire or other emergency, would you have known how to get to the fire exits? Would you even have known whether to turn left or right out of your hotel room? If there had been an intruder in your room, would you have been able to escape to the ground floor without hesitation? Most hotel rooms have floor plans on the door indicating the emergency exits. Don't ignore them. An SAS operative would have this information committed to memory from the first moment. You should do the same. Make yourself situationally aware. If there's no floor plan, do a recce.

Your second priority is to check the locking mechanisms on the door. Engage all deadbolts and other locks and keep them locked while you are inside. If there is a door jam, use that (I always carry one in my luggage for this purpose). Don't rely only on security chains or other mechanisms that allow you to half-open the door to see who's there — as I say, they're very easy to break. You can buy portable door locks that are easy to carry and which fit into the strike plate of your hotel door. These can increase your security once you're inside your hotel room. I would particularly recommend these for lone female travellers.

Look at the furniture. Which of it can be moved? In the event of a hotel shooting, like those that occurred in Mumbai in 2008 and in Egypt in 2016, trying to escape the hotel is probably going to be too high-risk. Your only real option is to barricade yourself into your room. To do this, I'd go for a wardrobe first, then a bed. Once I'd got whatever furniture I could up against the door, I'd upend the mattress. Rounds from an assault rifle will easily rip through a hotel door, but any obstacles the round itself has to penetrate will make it lose energy – a mattress won't stop a round by itself, but it might catch it if the round has slowed down sufficiently. It will also offer some protection from shrapnel if your aggressor is armed with a fragmentation grenade, as the Tunisia beach shooter was. Once you've barricaded yourself in, you need to make sure you're well away from the trajectory a round might take through the door.

When you leave your room

Always leave the 'Do Not Disturb' sign on the outside of the door. The maids won't enter, and if intruders think there's someone inside, they're likely to move on.

In addition, I would always leave the TV and the lights on, so that it sounds as if you're in the room. In many hotels, you need to put your key card into a slot by the door in order for the lights and electricity to work. This is why you need two cards (see above): one to take with you, one to leave in the slot.

If you lose your hotel key or key card, immediately tell the hotel. It may have been stolen. Get the codes changed, or move to another room.

Be hyper-aware of other people in hotel corridors and lifts. A common trick is for a criminal to watch a hotel guest leaving their room. If they then see them eating in the bar or restaurant, they know the room is empty. If you have suspicions, ask for a room change. Try to avoid being in a lift with just one other person – especially if you're a lone female.

How to tell if somebody is entering your room

I always carry with me a tiny tube of superglue. This enables me to tell if somebody has entered my room. To do this, you remove a hair from your head. Put a tiny dab of superglue at either end. When you leave the room, stick the hair on the corridor side of the door, right at the bottom where it's out of sight, and with one end stuck to the door itself and the other stuck to the doorframe. If someone enters your room, the hair will have snapped or come unstuck.

You can also use this trick to tell if somebody has been going through your drawers or wardrobe.

RESPONSES TO A TUNISIA-STYLE SHOOTING

At the beginning of this chapter, I told you that I would explain certain possible responses to a Tunisia-style beach shooting. I don't want to make light of this. It would be trite of me to suggest that there are any easy responses to such a situation. When somebody is firing indiscriminately your survival is, to a certain extent, a matter of chance.

But you can improve your odds.

As you will discover further on in this book, your survival priority when it comes to a mass firearms incident is evasion. This is why familiarisation is so important when you're in an unfamiliar place. If I were to take my family to the beach, especially in an environment such as Tunisia, where I knew there was a small but real threat of terrorist activity, I would immediately consider my exit routes. This would be informed by the time I had spent studying the surrounding area. If I need to run, I want to know *where* to run. If I was trying to escape the beach, I wouldn't want to end up down a dead end. If I was in the hotel when a terrorist entered, I would want to know where the exits are. If I need to escape the immediate area, I don't want to find myself in a part of town where the atmospherics are threatening and I can't be sure of the sympathies of the local populace. I need to make fast, accurate decisions at a time of high stress and personal danger. I simply can't do this if I haven't first taken the time to familiarise myself with the area.

In the wake of the Tunisia beach shootings, some tourists said that, when they heard the gunfire, they assumed it was fireworks. Again, this is where a heightened level of awareness comes in. Nobody sets fireworks off during the day. While it's true that gunshot is an unfamiliar sound for most people, by far the most dangerous mindset in a world where terrorist threats are increasingly likely is an assumption that they won't happen. If a sound *could* be gunshot, you should always be aware of the possibility that it *might* be. I would always assume that it is.

If I hear gunfire, I take a moment to establish the direction from which it's coming. This is particularly important in urban locations where the sound can echo off the building walls. It sounds obvious, but it's crucial to move away from the gunfire and not toward it: a lot of people have been killed in combat situations by making this elementary mistake. See page 243 for more on this.

Strategically, if you encounter gunfire on a beach, your evasive tactic should be to move inland toward buildings. If you run along the beach or toward the water, you remain in open ground and you are an easy target. I certainly would not advise going into the water, because then you make yourself a slow-moving target. You can't stay underwater indefinitely, and the gunman knows you'll reappear not many metres from where you submerged yourself. This happened in the 2011 Norway attacks by the far-right terrorist Anders Breivik. Having exploded a car bomb in Oslo, he moved on to a lake at a nearby summer camp and opened fire on crowds of teenagers. Many fled into the lake, some of whom sustained terrible injuries, and one of whom drowned. They would have stood more of a chance by scattering into the woodland, rather than getting into the water.

In heading toward buildings in Tunisia, I would not have been able to avoid reaching the vicinity of the hotel, but I would probably not have headed back inside it: if attacks are made in tourist destinations, the hotels are going to be likely targets. Instead, I would head toward areas where the locals live, because in this instance they were clearly not the targets. However, I say this with the proviso that I would avoid areas where the locals may not be sympathetic toward foreigners (which is information I would have identified during my famil-iarisation of the area). If you need to hide, do so – see pages 171–2 for more on this.

I would also aim to be aware of the possibility of herding. This is a terror tactic whereby targets are tricked into fleeing to a certain area, only to find that it's booby-trapped or there are more aggressors waiting for them. One of the worst examples of this was the Warrenpoint massacre in Northern Ireland, when the IRA ambushed a Parachute Regiment convoy with a roadside bomb, and placed a second bomb in a gatehouse where they knew the soldiers would set up an incident command point. In my opinion, it is only a matter of time before the current crop of terrorists adopt these tactics.

Finally, a worrying tendency is emerging for people to start filming these incidents on their smartphones. They are so keen to get the money shot that they forget about their personal safety. Make no mistake: if you are in sight or even earshot of somebody with a firearm, you are in mortal danger. This holds whether you're in Tunisia, Egypt, Mumbai or London. Put your phone in your pocket and move away from those rounds. It's not worth risking your life for some likes on Instagram.

For more advice on how to act if you find yourself in a mass terror incident, see Chapter 16.

CHRIS RYAN'S HOLIDAY SAFETY DEBRIEF

- Follow Foreign Office advice, and think carefully about porous borders near holiday destinations.
- Make familiarisation with your new location an immediate priority. Know your exit routes, and which areas to avoid.

- Don't look like a tourist.
- Be extra-vigilant in taxis and hire cars.
- Remember that hotels can be magnets for criminals, and act accordingly.

10

STAYING SAFE IN A RIOT

Somewhere in the Democratic Republic of the Congo there lives, if he's still alive, an African man who once had himself a second arsehole ripped by a furious Chris Ryan. The reason? For putting me and my team in the path of a mob, at night-time, in a city blighted by state-sponsored riots. It was one of the most dangerous moments of my time with the Regiment.

The DRC was called Zaire back then, and it was under the control of the dictator Mobutu. The economy was crashing. The poor had nothing to eat. In the capital of Kinshasa, lepers would congregate at the back of the hospital where the corpses came out, so they could steal body parts to eat. Kids lay starving in the street.

Mobutu's solution was to allow his troops to raid and loot wealthy houses in Kinshasa – most of which were owned by ex-pats, who by now had all been shipped out. The army would enter these properties and steal all the furniture, white goods, TVs and paintings – anything of real value – then local civilians would move in and strip it literally down to the bare blockwork in a matter of hours.

The mob was getting a taste for it, and it became clear that the foreign embassies in Kinshasa were under threat. All non-essential staff and family members were sent back to the UK. Our intelligence had indicated that there was a specific threat against the British Embassy. I was part of an eight-man unit despatched to Kinshasa to protect the British ambassador and the embassy itself from the rioting locals.

Eight SAS guys vs thousands of starving rioters. We didn't like those numbers much. But the UK had recently spent millions on the new ambassadorial compound. I guess they didn't want to see their investment go up in smoke, and to be fair, the lives of UK nationals were at risk. It was only ever meant to be a three-day op. As it turned out, we were there for a month.

The compound was surrounded by a six-foot-high wall. It wouldn't be too difficult to scale from the outside, so our first job was to cover it with razor wire. At the heart of the embassy there was a strong room where all sensitive documents were stored and which also included a secure communications centre. If the rioters did try to come over the wall, our strategy was simple. Four of us would get the ambassador into the strong room. The rest of us would set up a firing line and start dropping the intruders.

The British Embassy was next door to the US Embassy, which was being protected by some of the lads from Delta Force. I knew a couple of them and we fell into conversation.

'If it comes to it,' one of them asked me, 'what's your escape plan?'

They looked at me with incredulity when I told them. We had a single inflatable Gemini boat. Trouble was, it had a hole in it. We had to pump it up every morning and evening. If we needed to evacuate Kinshasa, we'd have to open up the gates of the ambassadorial compound, get across the road, down an embankment and into perhaps the fastest-flowing river in Africa.

'Why?' I said. 'What's yours?'

The Yanks had been airlifted into Kinshasa in a Galaxy Starlifter. They'd taken the precaution of bringing with them a Black Hawk and two Little Bird choppers. If the Delta guys said the word, the choppers would be in situ within five minutes.

'What weapons have you got?' they asked me.

'MP5s and pistols,' I said. 'You?'

'M16s, pistols, Claymores, grenades, 66s, gas, smoke . . .' The list went on.

We knew we were under-equipped, of course. Before we'd left Hereford, we'd made it clear to the headshed that we needed more weaponry and ammunition to deal with a situation like this, but the Foreign Office had refused to let us take what we wanted. A few days later, the Delta lads came round to see me with a present of grenades, gas and various other bits and bobs. Then they said goodbye and good luck. They were pulling out. Kinshasa was too dangerous, even for them.

But we were still there.

The atmospherics were off the scale. You could sense the unrest on the street. It came in waves. The crowds would come up to the wall at various times of the day – usually whipped into a frenzy by the army looting a wealthy house nearby – and you could feel the potential riot flaring up. Then it would all ease off, until the next time.

One of the local embassy officials lived off-site in Kinshasa. One night, he came to us in floods of tears. He was obviously drunk. He told us he'd just heard that the mob was raiding his house. There were top secret documents there, he said. 'You have to get them out!'

We saddled up, jumped into a couple of Land Rovers and exited the compound, along with the embassy official. We moved stealthily through the streets of Kinshasa until we reached the vicinity of the official's house. We came to a halt about 400 metres from the place. It was pitch black. No street lights. But just on the edge of my hearing, I could sense a low-pitched humming noise. Like many voices in the distance.

I took out my night sight and surveyed the ground up ahead. Through the dull green filter of the night vision, I could see a crowd just beyond the official's house. Two to three hundred people. Maybe more. It was difficult to tell in the dark. My skin prickled. We knew what this mob was capable of, and we could sense that it was on edge. One thing was very clear: if the mob realised there were eight British soldiers only a few hundred metres away, they'd have been all over us. This was a violent situation waiting to happen.

My instinct was to get the hell out of there. I turned to our unit leader. 'Mate, don't risk it. If they see us approaching the house and this kicks off, we're fucked.'

He overruled me.

Six of us dropped down into firing positions, our weapons trained on the area around the official's house. If any of the mob approached, we'd have no option but to drop them.

The unit leader and one other guy in the team started toward the house with the official, holding their pistols at their sides. I knew that if any of the mob saw that they were armed, we'd have a contact situation. When a crowd is fired up like that, all you need is somebody to light the touch paper. That's when people start to die. So my pulse was racing as I watched the three of them approach the house and disappear inside.

We kept our weapons trained. My finger was resting on the outside of the trigger guard. The mob was in my sights.

Three minutes passed. It felt like three hours.

The official and my two SAS mates reappeared. The official looked like he was carrying a pair of trousers. No documents that I could see. They returned safely to the vehicles. We piled in and got out of there, burning it away from the mob and back to the compound.

'Did you get the documents?' I demanded.

My unit leader could tell I was fired up. That's why he lied to me at first. 'Yeah, we got them.'

'Show me.'

He couldn't, so he came clean. He nodded toward the official. 'The drunk bastard was just looking for his dog,' he said. 'He couldn't find it. All he came out with was that spare pair of trousers. There are no frickin' documents.'

So when we got back to the embassy compound and out of the vehicles, the drunk official got a piece of my mind. I didn't hold back. This idiot had put us into a situation that was more perilous than he could possibly know. It had been a dangerous game of bluff. If that mob had spotted us and our weapons, I'm not sure I'd still be here to tell the story.

The reason I was so angry was that we had been forced into a situation where we had to do everything wrong. We knew rioting was a possibility, and our strategy revolved around *avoiding* the mob as far as possible, and only fighting back if there was no other option. Only someone with a death wish puts themselves in the path of an angry crowd. Riots don't generally come out of the blue. When they occur, you must do everything possible not to put yourself into the battle zone. And make no mistake: a riot *is* a battle zone. You need to understand the field of conflict in order to take the correct evasive action.

PRE-INDICATORS

It's normally clear from local media that rioting is a possibility. Don't ignore warnings of social unrest on traditional or social media. Get away from the area in question if you can. Stay indoors if you can't.

I was once in Paris as a civilian with a French friend. We heard a booming sound in the distance. I thought it was some kind of carnival, but my friend had heard that sound before: it was riot police banging their shields. We got out of there. So: if you see, or hear, police units – or sometimes even military forces – being bussed into an area or forming up, remember that they're doing it for a reason. You really don't want to be caught between them and a rioting mob. Move away.

Similarly, if you see crowds of civilian personnel moving away from an area, you should do the same. Don't hang around to see what it is they are so scared of.

Even if the rioters are protestors for whose cause you feel genuinely passionate, I would advise that you stay off the streets and clear of the incident. My experience is that even peaceful protests for good causes have a habit of turning ugly. Find some other way of showing your support.

UNDERSTANDING RIOT POLICE TACTICS

It is important to understand what can happen in a riot. Police responses are often – rightly – very forceful. If you're caught up in a riot, your personal safety can also be at risk from the police response.

I learned a lot about this when I did riot training with the Mexican *Federales*. Different police forces will have slightly different tactics, but the principles will remain the same. The front line of riot police will interlink, protected by their riot shields, rather like a Roman legion. Behind the front line there will be snatch squads, armed with batons rather than shields. As the police line moves forward, the person in command will be identifying key figures among the rioters – the people organising the riot. When the police line comes up against these people, it will open up to swallow in these key figures, who are then dealt with – often very brutally – by the snatch squads.

In addition, the police will have certain other riot control methods to hand.

CS Gas

Sometimes called tear gas, this is a very popular riot-control agent. Contact with CS gas causes a severe burning sensation to the eyes, nose and mouth, and a burning sensation in the chest if you inhale it.

When I was in the SAS, we trained with another riot control agent called CR gas. It's a thousand times stronger than CS gas and wouldn't be used on the general public in the UK, but you might encounter it in other parts of the world. As part of our training, we would let CS and CR canisters off in a room, then walk in without a respirator. We would say our name, rank and number, which forced us to take a breath and ingest some of the gas, and remain in there for thirty seconds before exiting. Every single guy would be coughing their guts out and in extreme pain. This stuff is seriously nasty. CR especially will put you on the floor.

If you suspect that there is CS gas in the vicinity, cover your face with a handkerchief or T-shirt and evacuate immediately. If you get it on your skin, wash it off with soap and water.

Rubber bullets

These were first used against rioters in Northern Ireland. They are supposed to be fired at the ground, so that they ricochet up at the legs. In reality, they are often fired directly at rioters. They really hurt – it's like getting punched, hard. There are different types, and the hard plastic ones will leave a big old bruise on your skin. They generally won't kill you, although there have been fatalities from rubber bullets.

Water cannons

These might sound like a less brutal method of crowd control, but they're not. There have been reports of water cannons tearing protestors' eyeballs from their face. Often the water contains dye to mark the rioters for later identification. Riot police will focus their water cannons on the ringleaders – another good reason to avoid the areas being targeted by them.

Tasers

These are increasingly popular with law enforcement. They administer intense pain, and have been known to kill.

Attack dogs

In many parts of the world, riot police have attack dogs on long leashes. I suggest you stay well clear of them. They don't know the difference between a rioter and an innocent civilian, they will bite anything that crosses their path and they are extremely savage.

Live ammunition

Depending on which country you're in, this is not just a possibility – it's a likelihood. Certainly if you get caught in a riot in America, you can be pretty certain there will be live rounds going down. It's precisely for circumstances such as this that armed police *are* armed . . .

NO-MAN'S-LAND

In a riot, there will be two opposing lines: the police line and the rioters' line. The void in-between them – think of it as no-man's-land – is the most dangerous location during a riot. This is where you're at risk of missiles from the rioters – think rocks, bottles and even Molotov cocktails. It's also where the police are going to aim their CS gas canisters (see below) and the area where you'll be caught in the line of fire between water cannons, rubber bullets, tasers and live ammunition.

If you find yourself in this area, you have three options. Most desirable first:

- Move to one of the extreme sides of the no-man's-land. In an urban environment, this will likely lead you to a building. Force yourself along the line of the building, taking care not to get caught up with rioters smashing windows or looting. The building line will eventually lead to an exit from the area.
- Push through the police line. Approach it with your hands up and your palms open, so they know that you're not a rioter and you have no hidden weapons. Once you get past the police line, you'll probably be hustled quickly and abruptly to the rear. But don't underestimate how dangerous it is being close to the police lines.
- Push through the rioters' line. Their aggression will most likely be toward the riot police, but this is still high-risk. Push on through them until you're free of the riot area.

HIDING

If you can't get away from the riot, you have to hide. You can read more about hiding on pages 201–4, but in an urban-riot situation, you need to get into an office building or shop. (Office buildings are better, because they are less prone to looting.) Break in if you have to, but if you're smashing a window, do it out of sight of the police, or they will mistake you for a rioter. Hide at the back of the building, as far from the riot as possible.

If you're able to access the city's underground system, this can be a good place to head, because you can get on a train that will take you out of the riot area. It's possible that any CS gas will follow you down, but if it's going noisy at street level, I'd much rather risk this than exposure to the riot. CS gas is nasty, but it won't cause any lasting harm.

If there are riots near your home, you should stay in your (locked) house. A good strategy, however, is to put a sign on your door stating that the occupant of the house is armed (whether you are or not). It will deter rioters and looters. If your family are with you, barricade the doors. Get them to the first floor, into a safe room if you have it (see pages 94–5). Remember how to establish a choke point (see page 100).

IF YOU'RE IN A VEHICLE

First off: if you're driving in an urban environment and you see signs of people moving away from an area toward you, don't drive on thinking that you're safe in your vehicle. If you do, you're making a potentially fatal error. Turn around and don't take the risk.

If you find yourself in a vehicle in the thick of a riot, the temptation may be to use your vehicle to drive through the crowds. This would be a mistake, especially if you can't see the far side of the rioting crowd. If you drive toward them, the chances are that you'll run someone over, in which case the mob will attack you. And if you drive toward the police lines, they will probably open fire.

Instead, you must exit that vehicle immediately, with your family if necessary, and follow the advice above to get out of there on foot. Don't worry about damage to your vehicle. Cars can be replaced much more easily than lives.

STAMPEDES

Stampedes often happen during riots, but at other times, too. A terrorist incident at a pop concert or sports event will cause an immediate rush to the exits and it can be very dangerous. If you're caught in a stampede, you risk asphyxiation and broken bones.

First, try to stay on your feet. As soon as you hit the floor, your chances of being crushed increase and you lose your ability to control the situation.

If you're with your family, lock arms so that you don't get separated.

As always, if you're in an enclosed area, you must be aware of your exit routes. If a stampede occurs, however, you shouldn't necessarily immediately head for the exits – that's what everyone else will be doing. Make a quick situational assessment and decide if you wouldn't be better finding a safe place to wait out the rush. This would be some kind of obstacle that won't move with the force of the crowd – a car or statue, perhaps. Position yourself on the lee side of it, so you're not crushed by the oncoming mass of bodies.

If you have to move to an exit point, never move against the crowd, or even at right angles to it. You can't withstand that kind of force. It's more effective to move with it, but at a forty-five-degree angle, so that you're going with the momentum of the crowd but also manoeuvring yourself to its edge, where you can break free of the surge of bodies.

If you can, get to high ground – the roofs of buildings or the upper levels of a stadium or arena.

CHRIS RYAN'S RIOT SAFETY DEBRIEF

- Be aware of media reports of social unrest. Avoid protests, even if you feel passionate about the cause.
- Understand that riot police use brutal tactics to quell riots – you don't want to be at the wrong end of them.
- The most dangerous place in a riot is the open ground between the police line and the rioters' line.
- Hide.
- In a stampede, find objects to shelter behind. If you can't, move with the crowd, heading diagonally toward your exit point.

11

HOW TO FIGHT

Let me give you an example why it's a very bad idea to pick a fight.

I was in Hereford. A couple of Regiment mates and I decided to get a Chinese takeaway. We were on the first floor of the restaurant collecting our food and my mate Sam was paying for the meal. He had a load of money in his wallet, which three pointy-heads in the line behind us saw. They decided they'd like to relieve my mate of his dosh.

The pointy-heads followed us as we carried our white plastic bags of Chinese food down to the ground floor. Then they confronted us. One of the lads fronted up to Sam. 'I want your wallet,' he said.

Before my other mate and I even had a chance to think, Sam smashed his bag of food into the lad's face. Red-hot chop suey exploded all over his skin. By the time I'd bent down to put my own bag of food on the ground, Sam had floored two of the pointy-heads and my other mate had floored the third. Two of them were knocked out. Sam bent down and removed the third guy's wallet. He helped himself to the contents and told the lad he was paying for our evening meal. Then we went on our way.

If the pointy-heads had been clever, they'd have sized us up before picking a fight. They'd have seen that Sam had a set of shoulders on him like cannonballs, fists like a miner's shovel, a broken nose and scars along his eye line from his career as an ABA boxer. The signs were there – they just didn't know how to read them.

But even if they *had* known how to read them, they'd have been playing a high-risk game. Fights are inherently unpredictable. Any one of us could have been carrying a knife, or even a gun. Those pointy-heads were risking a hell of a lot for the sake of a few notes.

Fighting should always be a last resort. I feel pretty confident handling myself, but I would never start a fight if I didn't have to. Moreover, if I had the option to run from a conflict situation, I would always do that. I urge you to do the same.

Sometimes, however, you can't run. Sometimes you are already in a conflict situation, and your only choice is to fight back.

How do you know if that moment has come? Your attacker's face will be fixed on you and they'll be moving toward you at speed. Their fists may be up. Either that, or they'll be shouting threatening abuse at you. This means the conflict situation has started. If you can't escape, you have to fight. Now, your safety and your life depends on your ability to attack.

In these situations, the coin is flipped. If you are in a position where you *have* to fight, it's critical that your actions are fast, shocking, brutal and above all effective. This is not the time for half-measures. All fighting is a risk. These are not playground punch-ups. Real fights expose you to the potential of being severely, even mortally wounded. Ineffective fighting makes you less safe, because it antagonises your aggressor and encourages them to be more brutal toward you.

Fight to win, or not at all.

Here's how.

FORGET THE MOVIES

You're not Bruce Lee. Nor am I. If you want information on martial arts and fancy self-defence manoeuvres, you've come to the wrong guy.

When the SAS respond to a situation, they are armed. Not just with firearms, but also tasers (if it's only a hard arrest), batons, grenades and gas. We're not on site to impress everyone with our punching skills. We don't want a fair fight. We're there to dominate the situation completely, using every tool we can to our advantage.

The trouble with unarmed, hand-to-hand combat is that it takes several lessons a week, every week, to become fluent in it and maintain your skills. For most people, that's unrealistic. So, although you won't be in possession of guns, tasers, batons, grenades or gas, I want you to take away some of the SAS mind-set when it comes to dominating a combat situation completely. We're going to learn how to fight dirty.

FIGHTING IS A NUMBERS GAME

Most of the time, when the Regiment enter a contact situation, they go in mob-handed. To put down an aggressive person, you want numbers on your side. It's the best way to dominate the situation.

But there is a flip side to this. If you're on your own and your aggressors substantially outnumber you, it means you have no realistic chance of overcoming them. The advice that follows holds for one-on-one conflict situations. If you are set upon by a group of aggressors, don't imagine that you can take them all out. They'll murder you. Get to the ground. Adopt a foetal position and cover your head and neck with your arms. This will help you to protect your chest, abdomen and vital organs in the beating that follows. Do everything you can to avoid blows to the head.

DON'T EXPECT ANY HELP

Stander-by apathy is the rule, not the exception.

I once filmed a TV programme in which I was done up to make it look as if I'd been severely beaten. I was lying in the gutter, looking a total mess, telling passers-by that I'd just been mugged and asking for help. Most people simply walked past, or even stepped over me. In all the time I was lying there, only one person – an Italian lady – offered me any help.

By contrast, as we were filming, two guys walked past and noticed that I was still wearing my watch. They were standing right next to one of the crew. One of them said to the other: 'That geezer's still got his watch on, let's do him.' When the crew member pointed out that we were making a film, they legged it.

The point is this: most people will avoid you if you look like you're in trouble. Some people will try to take advantage of it. You can't rely on anyone. Your safety is up to you.

SHOCK AND AWE

When a Regiment team storms a building or performs a hard arrest, it is very sudden, very noisy and very violent. There is a reason for this. That level of shock and awe is completely terrifying to somebody who hasn't experienced it. It makes them freeze. It stops them thinking clearly. It makes them much easier to dominate. I want you to learn from this. Sudden, surprising, violent action is your friend. Don't give any warnings. Don't circle around them trying to look threatening. Don't try to make them fear you with verbal abuse. If you have to fight, strike first and strike hard. Surprise them. Scare them. Scream loudly – this will make you appear a lunatic (which is what you want) and make your aggressor worry that other people might come to help. In both military and civilian conflict situations, a little shock and awe goes a very long way.

COMMIT YOURSELF

There's an old saying: You should never start a fight, but you should always finish one. Once you're committed to a conflict situation, it is essential that you see it through and win, up to the point that your opponent is completely incapacitated, or you're in a position to make your escape.

You cannot be squeamish. There may be blood. Broken bones. Screams. (Some of these may be yours.) If your opponent seems hurt, that is a sign to *increase* the violence of your actions and finish the job, not to step back. Wounded animals are very dangerous.

TARGET YOUR OPPONENT'S MOST VULNERABLE SPOTS

Kicking somebody in the shins or beating their forearms is *never* going to win you a fight. You need to target the most vulnerable, easily wounded parts of their body. The parts of the body that will really put them out of action if you attack them. In practice that means the eyes, the throat, the face, the neck and the genitals.

WEAPONS ARE EVERYWHERE

I'm not talking guns and knives. I'm talking bottles, rocks, fire-extinguishers, even the contents of a woman's handbag. In a fight, you must use anything close by to give you an advantage. This is especially true if your opponent is bigger, stronger and fitter than you. And particularly if you are a lone woman fighting a male attacker.

What you use as a weapon will depend on your environment, but here are a few examples to get you thinking in the right way:

- *Bottles*. Hold the bottle by the neck and smash the base. You now have a very effective weapon for glassing someone in the face.
- *Windows and mirrors*. Break them and grab a shard of glass. You can use this to slash someone.
- *Pens*. These make excellent stabbing weapons. Go for the eyes and throat.

- *A comb.* These can slash and tear the skin.
- *A rock*. If you violently smash a rock into someone's head a few times, they'll soon be on the ground.
- *A nail file.* This makes an excellent stabbing weapon.
- *A small can of hairspray*. In parts of Europe and the US, it is legal to carry cans of pepper spray for self-defence, and I would always encourage my daughter to do that where it's allowed. Where it *isn't* allowed, a small can of hairspray, squirted into an aggressor's face, will hurt and temporarily blind them.
- *A fire extinguisher*. Sprayed in the face of an aggressor, or used as a bludgeon or projectile.
- *Keys*. Good for stabbing in the face and eyes.
- *A belt*. For strangling.
- *Hot liquids.* Thrown straight in the eyes of an aggressor.

Often, just the process of you grabbing a weapon will make an attacker think twice. I saw a guy in a bar shout threatening abuse at another customer, only for the customer to break a couple of bottles and scream 'bring it on' at them. His potential attackers fled. Making yourself look like an aggressive, well-armed nutter can go a long way.

DON'T PUNCH

Punching is a real skill. It's all about twisting from the hips and pushing your weight in the right direction. For it to be effective, you need to spend time on a punching bag. If you haven't learned and practised how to punch, you'll be weak-wristed and won't land anything with the ability to stun.

It is much more effective to use the heel of the hand in a slapping or pushing motion. It you swipe the heel of your hand sideways against your opponent's chin, they'll feel like their jaw has just been broken (and it might have been). If you push the heel of your hand up into your opponent's nose, you have a good chance of breaking it and it will definitely be an agonising shock.

There are a couple of exceptions to this rule. If you can go in at the side and land a closed-fist punch in the lower back around the area of the kidney, you will wind your opponent to the point of incapacitation. A punch to the solar plexus will have a similar effect. In both these instances, you make your punch much more effective if the middle knuckle of your third finger is protruding from your closed fist.

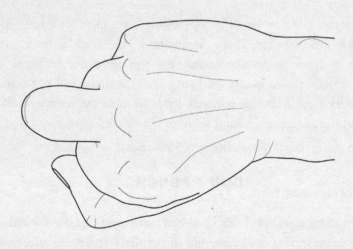

SOME AGGRESSIVE ATTACKING MOVES

Leave martial arts and intricate hand–to–hand combat skills to the pros. Instead, fight dirty to win fast.

Go for the eyes

Stabbing an opponent's eyes, or pressing your thumbs into their eye sockets, will quickly put them down. This is a very effective move if you're being throttled. Slide your arms up through your attacker's, grab the sides of his head with your palms and gouge your thumbs into his eyeballs.

Go for the ears

Ears are easily grabbed and very sensitive to pain. If you can seize your opponent's ear, yank it as hard as you can, as if you're trying to rip it off.

Go for the throat

A solid blow to the throat will knock anyone down. Aim to crush their larynx – it will put them out of the game.

Go for the genitals

If you can get close enough, or if you're in a grappling hold, a foot or knee hard in the genitals is debilitating. If possible, grab your male aggressor's testicles and try to rip them off. (Remember that it's the testicles rather than the penis that will cause extreme, debilitating pain.)

Headbutting

Nutting someone in the face is a powerful way of inflicting damage. However, remember that you are aiming to strike their nose area with your forehead. If you go forehead to forehead, you'll do yourself as much damage as you'll do them, and you might even knock yourself out.

Scratching

Women in particular, if they have long nails, should use them to dig into their aggressor's face. This is painful and disorienting. It also has the advantage of capturing their DNA under your fingertips in the event of an attempted sexual assault.

Stamping

If your opponent is on the ground, stamp with your heel into his face as hard as possible. This makes use of the large muscles in your legs, so you can apply a higher level of debilitating force than you can with your arms.

Biting

If you can, get part of your opponent's body between your teeth, but with the full intention of breaking through the flesh and bone. It will be blindingly painful for them.

CHRIS RYAN'S FIGHTING DEBRIEF

- The SAS don't want a fair fight. They want to dominate completely. You must adopt the same mindset.
- Use anything you can as a weapon. Fight dirty.
- Target the most vulnerable areas of the body: eyes, face, throat, neck, genitals.
- Don't be squeamish, and remember that ineffective fighting puts you in more danger.
- Don't punch: swipe with the heel of the hand.

12

STAYING SAFE ON AN AIRCRAFT

Aircraft are not dangerous in the way most people think they are. Your risk of crashing is low, as is your risk of terror-related incidents and hijacking.

However, they're not completely safe. When you put yourself on a commercial aircraft, you put yourself in a confined space with people you don't know and whose temperaments you can't predict. Nine times out of ten, it's not a problem. Occasionally it is, and your safety may well depend on knowing how to deal with and defuse certain situations. And of course, when things do go wrong on an aircraft, they go *very* wrong. In this chapter, I want to give you some solid advice about aircraft security, informed by my time training on aircraft, and explain how to deal with certain emergency situations.

AIRPORT SECURITY

Every time I go through airport security as a civilian, I never fail to be surprised by the complaints I hear from other travellers. I have the impression that some people feel that the removal of your belt or the checking of your bags is too high a price to pay for ensuring your safety on an aircraft. I don't have much time for this point of view. The security measures undertaken at major airports have a demonstrable effect on safety in the air. My advice is to check in advance of your flight what you can and can't take on the aircraft, and don't try to argue with a security official who asks you to remove your shoes. You won't get anywhere.

However, please don't imagine that all airport security is as effective as Heathrow Terminal 5. I've been through plenty of African airports where travellers' luggage had been piled up without any surveillance, so that passengers can remove − or add − anything to it that they want. Give me a few extra minutes in the security queue any day. Also, don't kid yourself that airport security is infallible. On the day of 9/11, my daughter was flying home from Hungary after a camping trip. She inadvertently packed a sheath knife in her hand luggage. It wasn't noticed.

WHERE TO SIT ON AN AIRCRAFT

If you hit the internet and research which is the safest seat on an aircraft, you'll find all sorts of advice, most of which I would ignore. Your safety on an aircraft is defined not by your seat number, but by your situational awareness, as I will explain below.

That said, when I'm booking a flight there are certain seats that I avoid. It might sound counterintuitive, but those seats are in the rows on either side of the emergency exits. In the unlikely event of a hijacking situation, there is a good chance of special forces intervention. In order to gain access to the aircraft, the SF team will most likely breach the aircraft through these doors using high explosives. When I trained to do this with the SAS, we learned to accept that, in this situation, the people sitting in the adjacent rows would most likely be killed. Sure, you get a bit of extra legroom. Whether you think that's worth the extra risk is your call.

SAFETY ANNOUNCEMENTS

We've all heard the captain tell us how important it is to listen to the pre-flight safety announcement. I reckon almost everyone ignores it. So let me try to explain to you why ignoring that announcement is a really terrible idea, by telling you about three different SAS training exercises I underwent.

The first was when I was training with the guys one day at Pontrilas Army Training Area in Hereford. We were simulating a hostage rescue, which involved inserting from a Puma helicopter. As the Puma swerved into the training area, it banked too hard. The engine tone became more high-pitched. The soundproofing fell from the sides of the chopper. And the Puma came crashing down.

We were lucky. There was a ditch running alongside the road where we crash landed. The spinning blades turned into the ditch rather than hitting the ground. The aircraft bounced and the pilot managed to get it stable and then on to the ground. The chopper was written off – its tail section had snapped off – but thankfully everyone survived.

In the moment of that crash-land, every man experienced intense sensory overload. Imagine it. The aircraft is no longer upright, panic sets in, you have a moment of confusion as to where your exit routes are, and have very little time to make any decisions about your own personal safety. You're relying on what you know, not on what you can work out in the heat of the moment.

It's the same when you perform helicopter underwater escape training. You're strapped into a helicopter simulator and lowered – upside down and in darkness – into a swimming pool to simulate a crash in water. You regularly see people panicking, forgetting their emergency drills, not knowing when to unbuckle or where the exits are. It's frightening and confusing.

The third exercise I want to tell you about is one where we simulate an emergency situation on board an aircraft. To do this, we would fill a 747 with a crowd of two hundred students. We would divide them into three groups and give the members of each group a different coloured bib – yellow, red and green. One of us would privately tell one set of students that if, when the exercise began, they exited the aircraft before the others, they'd all receive a £20 bonus. The only proviso was that they couldn't mention this to any of the other groups. However, each group was told the same thing. When the exercise started, this meant we had swarms of students fighting each other to get out, climbing over the seats and pushing themselves aggressively down the aisles. We did this to simulate the mass panic that occurs when frightened people want to get off an aircraft. Trust me: it's not pretty. That wave of people stampeding through the aircraft is almost unstoppable.

Here's what I want you to take away from these three examples. When there is an emergency on an aircraft, your ability to make fast, effective decisions is severely compromised. There will be mass hysteria. It might be dark. You might be upside down. You might be injured. You will be scared.

So think again. Do you really want to stare at your phone while they're doing the safety announcements? Or do you want to check exactly where your nearest exit is? Do you really want to snooze? Or do you want to work out which direction your exit will be if the aircraft skids on the runway and turns upside down?

I've been on hundreds of aircraft. Civilian, military, in peaceful countries and in war zones. I *always* orientate myself properly when I get on to a flight. There's a saying in the military: train hard, fight easy. It means that you want your responses in an emergency situation to be second nature. That's what you're doing when you apply yourself to the safety announcements on a flight.

DISRUPTIVE PASSENGERS

Up until now, I've been advocating that we avoid conflict situations wherever possible in order to stay safe. However, I take the view that our responses to threatening situations on aircraft should be slightly different to our responses in other environments. Aircraft are enclosed spaces. When you're on a plane, it's not possible to escape or to move yourself from the potential field of conflict. With one exception, as I shall explain further in this chapter, it is incumbent on those who have the capability to nip any abusive and aggressive behaviour in the bud before it has a chance to escalate. As soon as we allow people to start running amok and assaulting others on aircraft, we risk the situation becoming much worse for far more people. There is a time to back off and there is a time to dominate. This is the latter.

I'd been diving in Sharm el Sheikh, Egypt and was now on my flight home. There were five young men in the seats in front of me. It was clear from the moment we boarded that they were going to be trouble.

As I was strapping myself in, an air stewardess came up to talk to them. 'I was on the same flight as you lot coming out,' she said. 'You were smoking. I've told the captain you're on board. If you use the toilets to smoke on *this* flight, we'll get diverted and you'll be arrested. Is that understood?'

One of the guys gave her the evil eye. I could tell he didn't like being spoken to like that.

As soon as we were in the air, the ringleader was kneeling up on his seat, holding court for his cronies. The air stewardess arrived to find out who had paid for in-flight meals. The ringleader demanded a vegetarian meal. When the air stewardess asked if he'd booked it, he said, 'No, but I still want one.'

She told him he couldn't have it. So this guy picked up a can of Coke and threw it at her. The can hit the back of her head.

The air stewardess turned to me. 'Did you see that?' she asked. 'Will you make a statement?'

I told her I would. I went to the back of the aircraft with her and made the statement. When I returned to my seat, the guys were giving *me* the dead eye. I could tell I was going to have problems with them.

A little later, the air stewardess came past with the bar service. One of the guys elbowed her aggressively in the thigh. I jumped up from my seat and confronted him. 'You'd better stop it,' I told him, 'otherwise we'll be diverted and I want to get home.'

The ringleader stood up. 'And what are you going to do about it?'

We were face to face. 'Fucking try it,' I breathed.

I was ready to put this low-life out of action. But I would much prefer that he backed off of his own accord. I looked over my shoulder. Several well-built guys were studiously avoiding looking up. I pointed to one of them. 'You,' I said. 'Get up here and help us.'

He did as I asked, albeit reluctantly. And once I had one reinforcement, a few of the others joined us. All of a sudden, numbers were on my side. I could see the ringleader assessing his options. We were in a contained area. He had no escape routes. He clearly wasn't used to anyone calling him out for this kind of behaviour and now the situation wasn't what he thought it would be. He backed down and took his seat again.

We started our descent into the UK. The captain told everyone to strap themselves in. As the air stewardess passed by again, however, the ringleader elbowed her in the leg for a second time. I confronted them again. Told them to back off. Made it clear that I wasn't going to stand for his bullshit.

Again, the situation died down. We landed. The captain came over the loudspeaker. 'Everyone stay in your seats,' he said. 'The police are about to board.'

The police arrived and arrested three of the gang. As the passengers stood up to disembark, I found myself flanked by the remaining two. One of them was a very big lad. 'I'm going to do you when we get outside,' he told me.

If you've read this far, you'll know that my advice is always to avoid a fight if you possibly can. Flanked by these two thugs as we made our way to passport control, I was pretty sure that avoidance wasn't going to be possible. They stuck close to me as we zigzagged up to passport control. I sized them up, evaluating my options. If I had to enter a conflict situation with them, I would. And I would win.

The big fella reached passport control before me. He started patting himself down, looking for his passport. Only then did he realise that one of his mates who had been arrested was carrying it. The passport control officer didn't have much sympathy. 'You sit over there,' he said. 'When the police release your friends, you can come through.'

I don't know what annoyed him more – being delayed or seeing me sail through passport control while he was helpless to do anything. I guess he didn't know he'd been given a get-out-of-jail card – I'm fairly certain I could have put those two on the floor without too much trouble. I gave him a smile and a wink as I entered the UK and went on my way.

It was only subsequently that details of IS training camps in Egypt came to light. I'm not saying that was definitely the reason these jokers had been to Egypt, but put it this way: they were fit, motivated, aggressive, unpleasant guys. I don't think they had been visiting the pyramids.

193

The point of this story is to illustrate that on a flight, when everybody is cramped together, sometimes you can't be a bystander.

Be aware of the passengers around you. I always do a quick recce of everyone in the vicinity of my seat. I'm not only trying to identify the potential trouble-makers. I'm also looking for guys who I think might provide useful backup in a contact situation.

If somebody seems to be drinking too much, and especially if they've brought their own supply on board, I would inform the cabin crew. Nine times out of ten, that kind of behaviour will end badly. If the cabin crew are aware, they can refuse to serve them any more booze from the trolley, or issue a warning if necessary.

If a passenger strikes out at a flight attendant, or two or more passengers start fighting among themselves, or if someone has clearly lost the plot on account of alcohol or drug consumption, my opinion is that it is the duty of other passengers to subdue them and, if necessary, restrain them. This is not something the cabin crew can necessarily do by themselves.

Be a leader. If the cabin crew look like they're having difficulty with a passenger, ask if they need any help. If they do, there will always be several guys on the plane (or women, if the disruptive passenger is a woman) who will be in a position to help out – but they'll probably only do it if you lead the way.

In the incident above, the threat of action was enough to subdue the disruptive passengers. This won't always be the case. You may have to restrain them yourself. To do this, you first need to get them on the ground. This is a numbers game: get several guys to bundle the troublesome passenger to the ground, keep hold of both his arms and both his legs, and don't release him. Try to get him listening to you. If he won't, you can use necessary force. Most aircraft carry restraints to keep disruptive passengers in their seats. It will be up to the aircraft's captain to decide whether a passenger should be physically restrained.

If you're having trouble keeping a disruptive passenger subdued, I want to give you two tips. Both of these require the use of a pen, or anything hard and similarly shaped:

- Stand behind the passenger. Put the pen under his nose, holding both ends. Pull from behind. This inflicts extreme pain and will force anyone to be compliant.

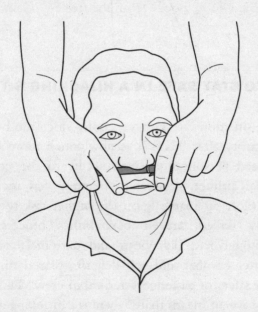

- If the disruptive passenger has grabbed someone and won't let go, put your pen against the top of his wrist and tuck your fingers under his wrist. Squeeze hard. It will hurt and he'll let go.

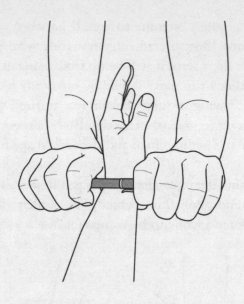

HOW TO STAY SAFE IN A HIJACKING SITUATION

Hijacking situations are rare, especially since the bolstering of airline security after 9/11. It is now much more difficult for unauthorised personnel to gain access to the cockpit of a commercial airliner, passenger screening has increased, and there are more air marshals on the higher-risk routes. (These are highly skilled, armed plainclothes officers, adept at recognising terrorist behaviour and extremely proficient in close-quarter combat and self-defence, placed on aircraft to ensure the safety of passengers and cabin crew.) This is all good news. However, it means that if there *is* a hijacking attempt, it is likely to be carried out by very well-organised, highly moti-vated criminals. With this in mind, I want to give you a few tips as to how I would react in a such a situation.

As soon as you become aware that your aircraft is being hijacked, you must make an assessment: is this a hostage hijacking, or is it a suicide mission? This will inform your response. If it seems to be a hostage hijacking, where the aim of the hijackers is to get the aircraft on to the ground so that they can extort a ransom or achieve political ends or publicity, my general advice would be to go with it. I said above that there is one rare circumstance when you shouldn't nip a disruptive incident on an aircraft in the bud. This is it. Your chances of survival are pretty good in this situation. Be aware, though, that once you're on the ground, there may be a special forces response. Remember the advice above about sitting adjacent to the entrances of the aircraft.

If it becomes clear that the hijackers have murderous intent – they mean to kill everyone on board and/or use the aircraft as a 9/11-style weapon – you must do everything you can to overpower them. If you don't, you're dead, so any risk you can take is worth it.

The advice above about subduing and restraining personnel on aircraft all holds. Lead the attack – if you don't, there's a chance nobody else will – and understand that your best strategy is to significantly outnumber the hijackers. A 4:1 ratio is the best, because it means there is one person to restrain each limb.

Be very aware, however, of the possibility of sleepers – accomplices among the passengers watching and waiting to deal with any response that you might try to initiate. As always, this is where your situational awareness comes in. There are no fool-proof ways of identifying sleepers until they identify themselves, but being aware of their possible presence will help you respond if they do.

In Chapter Eleven, you'll have read some tips about applying violence when it is necessary. Follow them without hesitation and with all the force you can muster. If you've managed to restrain a hijacker, you need to search him or her for the presence of explosives. If you find them, there will usually be a hand-held detonating device: you must make sure the hijacker cannot access it. Move him or her away from the area around the wings – this is where the fuel is generally kept on an airliner, and so is the worst place for a detonation.

As well as restraining a hijacker, I would always gag and blindfold them, too. This stops them being able to communicate with each other or with any sleepers.

CHRIS RYAN'S AIRCRAFT SAFETY DEBRIEF

- Airport security might be a drag, but it's important.
- The best emergency-situation advice on an aircraft doesn't come from me, it comes from the cabin crew. Listen to their safety briefing.
- Understand that aircraft emergency situations are frightening and disorientating. Time spent making yourself actively aware of your exit routes is never wasted.
- If there are disruptive passengers, support the cabin crew and be prepared to take the lead and restrain them if necessary.
- Hijacking situations are rare. If it's a hostage situation, go with it. If your life, and that of your fellow passengers, is under threat, do whatever it takes to put the hijackers down.

13

HOW TO RUN AND HOW TO HIDE

Much of the advice in this book centres around the importance of knowing when to run and hide. So far, I haven't told you *how* to do this.

Escape and evasion is a crucial military skill. Don't confuse it with cowardice. If you've made a dynamic assessment of a battlefield or a threatening situation, and you've established that your personal safety requires you to move yourself away from the threat, you must do this immediately. But you must also be aware that running and hiding are not random acts of flight. This isn't a child's game of hide and seek – this is you potentially keeping yourself and your family alive and unharmed.

I feel qualified to talk about this because I hold the record for the longest escape and evasion in SAS history. This happened when I trekked across Iraq to the Syrian border in the wake of the Bravo Two Zero mission. I was able to do this because of the training instilled in me by the SAS from day one. Be in no doubt: these are core skills for a special forces soldier.

HOW TO RUN

Sometimes running may be your natural instinct. Other times, you might freeze in terror – the old rabbit-in-headlamps scenario. A good way of overcoming this freeze response is to tell yourself that by running, you are taking positive steps to ensure your safety. You're not running away from danger, you're running *to* safety. You should also understand that fear can be your best friend – not least because the adrenaline rush it provides can make you run faster.

Once you've started running, avoid looking back. It slows you down and it increases your chances of tripping or hitting an obstacle. Focus on what is ahead of you, not what's behind you.

You will need to make an assessment about how much noise to make. If there are other people around and you want to alert them to your predicament, or get them to stand ground with you, scream your head off. If it's just you and your pursuer in the vicinity, keep quiet: the more noise you make, the more you identify your position. Shouting is also very tiring. Keep your breath for the more important business of getting away.

Don't run blindly. Although you'll be scared, you must try to maintain your situational awareness, so that you can use your environment to its best advantage. Scan ahead as you run. Can you see any side streets or junctions? It's a good idea to change direction as often as possible when you're running, as it increases the chance of your pursuer losing you. Sudden direction changes are also effective if your pursuer is very close behind: it keeps you in control and it increases the chances of your pursuer losing their footing. Just ensure that, if you make sudden changes in direction, you do so without slowing down and allowing your pursuer to make up ground.

Scanning ahead and being aware of your environment also ensures that you're on the lookout for items you can use as incidental weapons to fight your pursuer if necessary. Whether or not you choose to do this will depend on your situation. Are you faster than your pursuer? Keep running. Do you think they're going to catch up with you? Prepare to enter a conflict situation. Look for weapons, obstacles to throw in their path, and cover.

In general, you should try to run toward crowds or into shops or other inhabited areas, where you can get help or at least alert others. If you can't do this, or if your attacker is armed, or if he or she is fitter than you and you're tiring, it may be that you need to hide.

HIDING

Hiding is a very important skill in the SAS. A big part of a Regiment man's job is surveillance, often behind enemy lines. We might, for example, need to establish an LUP – a lying-up point – from which we can observe and report upon enemy movements. If we're going to do this, our lives and the success of the mission depend upon us not being seen. So, one of the most important lessons we – or indeed any other military personnel – learn is how things *are* seen.

How things are seen

There is a mnemonic – the 6 S's – to remind us how and why things are seen:

- *Shape*. If a human stands on the brow of a hill, it is completely obvious that it's a human even from a very long distance. The shape is unmistakeable. But if that human were to crouch down and maybe tuck his head into his arm, although he would be visible from a long distance, he wouldn't necessarily be identifiable.
- *Silhouette*. Whenever a shape is contrasted against a background of solid colour, it draws the eye. Let's go back to our human on the brow of the hill. He is silhouetted against the worst possible background: the sky. If he puts himself instead against a background of broken up, uneven shapes – trees, buildings, hedges – he is much more difficult to see.
- *Surface*. If the surface of an object has a different texture or reflectivity to its background, it's more likely to be seen. For example, skin – especially white skin – shows up against most backgrounds. That's why soldiers sometimes cover it with mud, if they don't want to be seen. When putting in an LUP, an SAS soldier will always be very aware of objects that might reflect light. Reflections can be unnoticed close up, but seen from miles away.
- *Shadow*. When the sun is out it can cast a shadow, which reveals an object that might otherwise be hidden. If an SAS soldier is putting in an LUP, he will always choose the north side of a slope, if possible, so that he remains in shadow and so doesn't cast one.
- *Spacing*. In the natural world, and to an extent in urban environments, objects tend not to be regularly spaced out. Regular spacing draws the eye.
- *Sudden movement*. You can be perfectly camouflaged, ticking all the above boxes. But if you move suddenly, you'll be seen. If you want to conceal yourself, you must keep very still.

A thorough awareness of the 6 S's will help you with your site selection when you hide. In an emergency situation, you're going to have to think fast, and you may not be able to mitigate against some of these factors. The more you can, however, the more likely you are to stay hidden.

The most important SAS technique when hiding

If a Regiment soldier needs to hide, he will always prioritise a location that other humans would rather avoid. This can be unpleasant.

Some years ago, I did a TV show called *Hunting Chris Ryan*, in which I had to escape and evade a hunter force of SF soldiers in various different environments. During one of these expeditions in Honduras, I laid up in a mangrove swamp that had live sewage running through it. I knew, even though I was being chased by SF personnel, that they would avoid wading through swamps filled with Honduran shit. When I finally extracted myself from the swamp, my legs were covered with blisters and sores from the lice and other insects crawling around in there. But I did evade capture.

If I was trying to evade an aggressor in an urban environment, I would be looking for skips, derelict building sites, sewers, culverts, canal-system tunnels, underneath motorway bridges, railway embankments. If I came across a large refuse site, I would have lucked out – especially if it smelt particularly bad. I'd get in there among the rats and the scavenging birds, knowing that I can probably hide in that location for as long as necessary – other humans are unlikely to come close.

If my environment was suitable, I would get myself into thick, thorn-filled bushes. If it hurt, I'd be doing something right.

Exit routes

When choosing a place to hide, don't box yourself in. Even if it's the best hiding place in the world, there's a chance someone will come across you by chance. Think: what will you do then? You always want to be able to escape your hiding place if you need to. (The exception to this is if you are hiding in a safe room that a predator can't access.)

BRAVO TWO ZERO

In practice, hiding places in emergency situations are seldom perfect. If there's a mass shooting and you secrete yourself in an unpleasant, smelly catering bin at the back of a restaurant, you're putting yourself in a location with no escape route. Hide in a relatively clean alleyway, you have an exit route, but you're placing yourself along a path that a predator is likely to follow.

You need to make in-the-moment judgements. When I escaped across Iraq, I had to travel by night and hide by day. To keep safe – to keep *alive* – I had to choose a number of different hiding places. Some were good, some were less good. I had to make a dynamic assessment at the time. To illustrate this, I'd like to describe some of these hiding places to you, so that you can start to build up a picture of what decisions need to be made when you're trying to hide.

Hiding place 1

My first hiding place was an Iraqi tank parking place or berm. This was a U-shaped elevation of earth, about two metres high, where a tank could park up and be hidden on three sides. I couldn't shelter inside the berm because the wind was blowing straight into it. Nor could I shelter on the lee side of it, because I'd have been exposed. My only option was to lie in the shallow indentations a tank had made.

This was a very poor hiding place. It was the only actual structure in the vicinity, which meant it was likely to attract people. If I had to escape, I would be in open ground. But there was no cover anywhere else nearby and it did the job.

Lesson learned: sometimes, when you're at risk, a poor hiding place is better than no hiding place.

Hiding place 2

My second hiding place was in a system of shallow wadis — dried-out river beds. This was quite a good place to hide. The wadi in which I hid kept me out of sight and offered some protection from the elements. It was also one of many, which meant that if somebody was searching for me, there would be a large number of almost identical choices for them to take. As it happened, however, I *was* discovered by a goat herder.

Lesson learned: even in good hiding places, you must be prepared for a chance discovery.

Hiding place 3

My third hiding place was also in a wadi. It was on a north-facing slope among some loose rocks. I knew that I would be in shadow all day as I hid, which was a positive. But I could still be seen from a distance. To mitigate against this, I buried myself into a hollow on the slope, and arranged loose rocks around me to break up the shape of my body. This dramatically improved the quality of the hiding place. Unfortunately, I was soaking wet, so being in shadow didn't help my personal comfort.

Lesson learned: don't expect your hiding place to be comfortable – the best way to do something is often the most difficult.

Hiding place 4

My fourth hiding place was on a rock face. Looking down the face from the desert floor I had seen a large crack. I'd known that if I could get in there, I would be invisible from above. Even though I had no exit route, it was a good hiding place, because it was difficult to get to, which meant other humans were likely to avoid it.

Lesson learned: finding a location that other humans will generally avoid trumps all the other factors when it comes to hideout site selection.

Hiding place 5

My fifth hiding place was a culvert – a tunnel under a road. It was about three metres high and a couple of metres wide, so it had obviously been built so that humans and animals could pass under the road. It was a terrible hiding place: a cold wind was blowing through it, and far from being a place humans would avoid, it was likely to attract them. And it did. I was forced to evacuate the culvert and secrete myself in a hollow in the ground for the remainder of the day, where I couldn't move around to keep myself warm, because movement would have made me obvious.

Lesson learned: be adaptable, and if your hiding place is compromised, move fast to evacuate.

Hiding place 6

My final hiding place was again a culvert. This time it was a better choice, though not perfect. The tunnel was one of three that passed under a busy six-lane highway. They were about the diameter of a 45-gallon drum. Two of them were clean. One was unpleasant and full of rubble. I chose the rubble-strewn one. It was a risk, because it meant I was boxed in at either end. But I was taking a calculated gamble that even if Iraqi forces searched the two clean culverts, they would avoid the dirty, rubble-strewn one.

Lesson learned: if you have the choice between a comfortable but less secure hiding place, and an uncomfortable but more secure hiding place, always prioritise security.

Ultimately, running and hiding often rely on a little good luck. But it's amazing how much luckier you get when you allow your escape and evasion to be proactive rather than reactive. An SAS man always tries to make good choices in an operational setting, rather than have decisions forced upon him. I'd encourage you to do the same if you or your family find themselves having to evade threats in everyday life.

CHRIS RYAN'S RUNNING AND HIDING DEBRIEF

- Use your adrenaline. It makes you faster and helps you think quicker.
- Run tactically. Apply sudden changes in direction and be aware of potential obstacles you can put in the way of your pursuer.
- Shape. Silhouette. Surface. Shadow. Spacing. Sudden movement.
- The more disgusting a location, the better it is as a hiding place.
- Always consider your exit routes.

14

INDENTIFYING AND
UNDERSTANDING FIREARMS

In Northern Ireland during the Troubles, two regular green army lads were driving through the Province when they stumbled across an IRA funeral procession. Not a great place for a British soldier to be. Sure enough, the crowd surrounded their vehicle and started trying to break in through the windows. One of the young soldiers had a Browning 9mm handgun. As the mob rocked the vehicle, he fired a warning shot into the floor of the car.

But the Browning 9mm has a flaw. The magazine-release button is on the left-hand side of the pistol. If you grab it and you're not thinking – and especially if you have big hands – you'll hit that button and the magazine will drop down about a centimetre. If you're not highly competent with it, you won't realise you've had a stoppage.

This is precisely what happened when the lad fired his warning shot. He squeezed the gun too tightly and inadvertently released the magazine.

One of the IRA men who was outside the car, banging on the soldiers' window, saw this. He had a good understanding of the Browning pistol – better than the young soldier, who wasn't fully competent with his weapon and didn't know his stoppage drills. The IRA man, on the other hand, knew that there wasn't going to be another round coming out of that pistol. He kept banging on the window until it smashed.

Both guys were dragged out. The IRA roughed them up and went through their wallets. They found a membership card for a video club in a place called 'Herford'. Herford was the location of the British Army base in Germany. But the IRA lads misread it as 'Hereford'. They thought they had two SAS men on their hands. Which meant the soldiers' fate was sealed. They were dragged from the area and executed. The IRA used the same Browning that had let them down in the first place.

I hope you or your family never encounter a situation where firearms are being used against you. If you do, you are of course in mortal danger. But if the story of the two young green army soldiers tells us anything, it is this: in a firearms incident, an understanding of the firearm involved can tip the balance.

In this chapter, I'm going to give you the low-down on the different types of firearms you're likely to encounter in an urban environment. Let me make one thing clear: this is *not* a tutorial on how to operate or fire a gun. I do not take the view that civilians need to know such information. Nor is it an exhaustive list of weaponry. We won't be concerning ourselves with rocket-propelled grenades, .50-calibre machine guns or any other type of firearm that you would probably only come across in a war zone.

Instead, we're going to look at four different categories of weapon: handguns, submachine guns, assault rifles and shotguns.

We are going to do this because an understanding of what these weapons are and how they are used might just be the difference between life and death for you and your family, if you should find yourself in a firearms incident.

HANDGUNS

For our purposes, we can divide handguns into two main types: semi-automatic pistols and double-action revolvers. From the point of view of the user, each has their advantages and disadvantages.

Semi-automatic pistols

The term 'semi-automatic' means that once one round is fired, the recoil generated by the expelled round ejects the empty cartridge case, loads the next round and cocks the hammer of the weapon. In layman's terms, this means that the user can fire multiple rounds in quick succession.

Semi-automatic pistols are magazine-fed. Each magazine usually houses twelve or thirteen rounds. The ability to house a relatively high number of rounds that can be discharged in quick succession, along with the weapon's concealability, is what attracts users to a semi-automatic, but they do have their disadvantages. They require a lot of practice to use effectively, and have a large number of working parts, which means more stoppages.

There is a simple way to see if a semi-automatic has had a stoppage. The actual barrel of the weapon is housed inside a moveable outer casing called the slide. Normally, you can't see the barrel. If you *can* see it protruding from the end of the slide, it means the gunman is experiencing a stoppage.

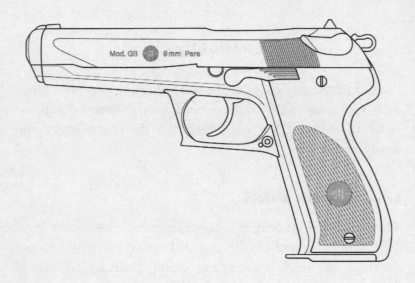

Double-action revolvers

Revolvers are so-called because they have a revolving chamber, which normally houses five or six rounds. They are called 'double-action' because there are two ways of firing them. You can pull back the hammer, in which case you are on a hair trigger and the very slightest movement will fire the weapon. Because there is less movement, this method is more accurate for an aimed shot. Or you can simply squeeze the trigger, which will cock the weapon and fire it. This is less accurate, because there is more trigger motion.

Different revolvers have different barrel lengths. You might have a 6-inch barrel, or a 2-inch 'snubnose' barrel. The longer barrel is much more accurate and powerful. The shorter barrel is much easier to conceal.

Revolvers almost never experience stoppages. This is their principal advantage over pistols.

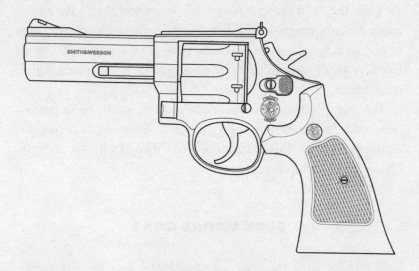

Both pistols and revolvers are hard to aim. During my time in the Regiment, I spent very many hours on the range learning how to fire these weapons accurately. I'd be confident of taking a headshot on a stationary target with a semi-automatic pistol at about forty feet. If it was a moving target, I'd go for a body shot first. On the other hand, most criminals or terrorists, despite being in possession of a pistol, will probably hardly ever have fired it. I'd be surprised if they could reliably hit a stationary target at more than ten to twenty feet.

This doesn't mean, of course, that there isn't a danger of stray rounds with a much longer range. The *effective* range of these weapons in the hands of an untrained gunman might only be twenty feet, but the rounds travel much further than that, the exact distance depending on the weapon. Compared to the other weapons in this chapter, however, they are probably the least effective in the hands of a criminal or terrorist, because they are the most difficult to get on target and they have a relatively limited range. In the hands of a terrorist, they are most often used for short-range assassinations at a range of one to five feet. But primarily they are designed for self-defence, rather than attack.

Terrorist groups across the globe are known to be in possession of a wide variety of handguns. They were used, for example, during the Parisian *Charlie Hebdo* attacks and the Orlando nightclub shootings.

SUBMACHINE GUNS

Submachine guns are designed to give the user the fire-power of a machine gun with the portability of a handgun. Soldiers would use them in close-quarter battle scenarios. Common varieties include the MP5, the Uzi and the Mag 10 (technically a machine pistol).

These weapons are magazine-fed. They are designed to fire the same cartridges you'd use in a handgun, but in larger quantities and at a much faster rate. So, while they remain compact and easy to conceal, you can operate them with a twenty- to thirty-round magazine. An MP5 will have a range of about 400 feet, although you'd be lucky to hit someone with an aimed shot at more than 200 feet.

Submachine guns can be set to semi-automatic, as with the semi-automatic pistol, or fully automatic. This means that the weapon keeps firing in a burst until you take your finger off the trigger. In semi-automatic mode, their effective range is similar to that of a handgun (though again, the rounds will travel much further than a terrorist or criminal will be able to aim them). Many variants have a retractable butt, so that they can be used to take aimed shots.

But ... criminals and terrorists generally choose submachine guns for their fully automatic mode. On automatic, the weapons become harder to aim accurately because, as with most weapons, they have a tendency to rise to the right in untrained hands when fired. But because of the furious rate of fire, they are mainly used to spray bursts of rounds, which are extremely deadly at close quarters.

For this reason, they are known as 'spray and pray' weapons. They are the firearm of choice for gangs performing drive-by shootings, but because of the untrained user's inability to aim the weapons properly, it's often the innocent bystanders who get killed in the crossfire, rather than the actual target. They are devastating in confined areas.

Submachine guns are prone to stoppages, especially if they're not clean and you're using cheap ammunition.

Terrorist groups are known to be in possession of submachine guns. They are ideal for attacks where a weapon must be easily concealed, yet still deliver a high rate of firepower on a target. But, as I've said, they're also the weapon of choice for many street gangs. An Uzi was used, for example, in a drive-by shooting in Harlesden, London in 2016.

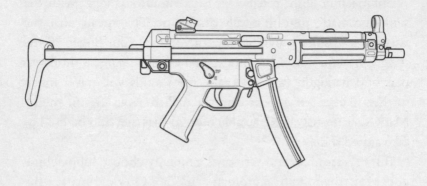

ASSAULT RIFLES

Like submachine guns, assault rifles can be set to semi-automatic mode or fully automatic mode (and some variants have settings that allow controlled bursts of a certain number of rounds). They are also magazine-fed. They differ from submachine guns in that they have much longer barrels and they fire higher calibre rounds. The most widely used assault rifle in the world, and probably the most popular gun ever, is the AK-47. They generally have thirty rounds per magazine.

Assault rifles have a much longer effective range than handguns or submachine guns. A trained marksman such as myself, if they were using their own weapon that had been properly zeroed in, would be confident about hitting a target with an aimed shot at 600 metres (and the rounds will be deadly beyond that). Even an unskilled shooter, however, would be able to get pretty close to target at 300 metres. They are prized by terrorists and militant groups, not only for their range and automatic fire ability, but also for the ability of the rounds to penetrate glass and even steel.

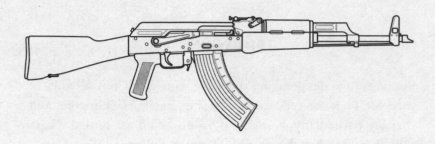

Although they are quite common in urban environments across the world, these are weapons of war. The damage done by an assault rifle's round, such as a 7.62 or a 5.56, is extreme. When they are used in civilian settings, they are devastating. And I knew a guy in the Regiment who, after serving in the first Gulf War, managed to smuggle an AK-47 back in to the UK. He subsequently left the Regiment to become a doctor. When he was in his fifties, he started dating an eighteen-year-old nurse. It was never going to last, and when she left him, this idiot went on the rampage with his AK. He found his ex in a pub and opened up on her. She was hit by ten rounds as she tried to escape. One of them blew her kneecap off. Another severed her arm. They caused catastrophic damage to her body, before he finally landed the shot that killed her.

Like pistols and submachine guns, assault rifles can be prone to stoppages. But they are the terrorist's weapon of choice. They were used during both the *Charlie Hebdo* and the Champs Elysées attacks in Paris, for example, as well as during the Tunisian beach attack and the Orlando nightclub shootings.

SHOTGUNS

Shotguns are designed for hunting. But that's not all they're used for. They are very easily available on the black market and they are particularly well-suited for unskilled marksmen. That's why they are often the choice of armed criminals.

Shotguns fire cartridges. The cartridges are normally filled with lead pellets. When the cartridge is discharged, the pellets spread out. At the end of the barrel of a shotgun is a choke. This tightens or widens the spread of the pellets. A wider spread can also be achieved by sawing off the end of the barrel – you've probably heard of a sawn-off shotgun. In a confined area, such a weapon is extremely effective. Fire a sawn-off into a room and everyone's going to get a piece of it.

There are shotgun cartridges that *aren't* filled with pellets. Some have a slug of solid shot – a single lump of metal that will make a hole in pretty much anything you fire it at. Certain anti-terrorist units are starting to use a specialist solid-shot round that will even penetrate Kevlar body armour and steel. It would be difficult for a criminal or terrorist to get hold of one of these, but not impossible.

The most common types of shotgun are break action, pump action and semi-automatic. A break-action shotgun has two barrels, either side by side or on top of each other. These are generally used for shooting birds or clay pigeons. A round is manually loaded into each barrel. When both are discharged, you 'break' the barrel (lever it down from the butt) to reload.

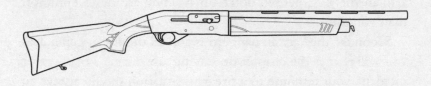

Pump-action shotguns have a single barrel and a sliding lever, which must be pumped to reload. Semi-automatics reload automatically when a cartridge is fired. It used to be the case that these types of shotgun were allowed a maximum of five cartridges in their magazine. That has now been limited to three and pretty much all registered shotguns will have been converted accordingly. Be aware, though, that it doesn't take the brains of an archbishop to reset these weapons. If you see someone with a single-barrel shotgun, assume three cartridges, but be prepared for five.

It is common for criminals to saw off most of the butt of a shotgun, as well as sawing off the barrel. This allows them to tie it to a cord or lanyard so that it can be slung over their shoulder and easily concealed under a coat.

Shotguns are more likely to be used by street criminals or amateur terrorist groups. A pump-action shotgun was found in the vehicle of the Champs Elysées shooter.

WHAT THE PRESENCE OF THESE WEAPONS MEANS TO A CIVILIAN

Firstly: don't believe that just because it's illegal to carry a firearm in the UK, people don't do it. They are more common than you think.

Secondly: they are all dangerous and all deadly. In general, as you will read in the chapter on staying safe during a mass terror incident, your response to a firearms situation should always be to get away from the gunman if possible, and to hide if you can't.

Now that we know a little bit about these types of weapon, however, we can use this information to give us the edge.

Handguns are short-range weapons and difficult to fire over long distances. This means you have a better chance of escaping a gunman armed with one of these if you run presenting a moving, zigzagging target. You should *never* do this if you can escape without entering the shooter's line of fire, or hide. But if these aren't options, use your knowledge of the weapon to make the best call.

Submachine guns are also difficult to fire, but their automatic capability means that unskilled people can spray and pray. Get low and take cover, and watch for stoppages and reloads.

Assault rifles have long effective ranges and the ability to pierce very solid structures. Again, take cover, but be prepared to bolster the walls and doors of your hiding place with whatever improvised ballistic shields come to hand. And again, watch for stoppages and reloads.

Shotguns are most deadly in confined spaces, where it is most important that you take cover. In open spaces, running might be an option if you can get enough distance. The shorter the barrel, the wider the spread, but the shorter the range. Expect only three rounds before a reload (but be prepared for five).

HOW TO SPOT A CONCEALED WEAPON

The easiest type of firearm to conceal is a handgun. These will most likely be secreted in a holster at the ankle, the waist, or across the chest. You might see a bulge where the weapon is located, but this will depend on what clothes the gunman is wearing. And to an SAS man, the bulge of the weapon is not necessarily the primary indicator that someone is armed.

An SAS man is comfortable with a weapon. We spend hundreds of hours training with them and we routinely use concealed weapons on urban ops. But while we are at ease carrying a firearm, most people are not. They appear uncomfortable when they walk. Their gait stiffens up. If you're aware of your surroundings and the people around you, that unusual gait is the first thing you're likely to notice. A bulge in the standard holster locations acts as confirmation.

Larger weapons are, of course, more difficult to conceal. On page 141, we discussed the gunman who opened fire on tourists on a Tunisian beach. He had his AK-47 hidden inside a beach umbrella. I'm certain that this would have been noticeable to a bystander paying proper attention. His hands would have been holding the stock of the weapon and the umbrella would have appeared heavier than normal. To the trained – or at least the observant – eye, it would have looked all wrong. As always, it's a question of being sensitive to things looking out of place. Why's that guy carrying an umbrella down the street? Where's its base? Does it match the other umbrellas on the beach? Large weapons are hard to hide. There will almost always be some indication of their presence.

If a criminal has tied a lanyard to a sawn-off shotgun and is secreting it under a coat, you'll notice that their arm will be pushed out somewhat. It will look awkward. And of course, their coat may be unseasonable, which should ring alarm bells anyway.

Finally, be aware that sometimes the best place to hide is in plain sight. If somebody in a crowd was walking with their handgun by their side, would you really notice it? This happens more often than you'd think, because gunmen know that the average joe probably doesn't have the situational awareness to notice it. By this stage in the book, I'm hoping that average joe isn't you.

You will find more information on how to act in the presence of armed personnel on page 243.

CHRIS RYAN'S FIREARMS DEBRIEF

- Know the difference between handguns, submachine guns, assault rifles and shotguns.
- Consider the gunman's effective range.
- Count the rounds if you can.
- Remember that unskilled gunmen often look nervous and uncomfortable when they're carrying a weapon.

15

STAYING SAFE IN A HOSTAGE SITUATION

If you are a UK national and you are taken hostage, either in this country or abroad, it will be the role of the SAS to rescue you. In fact, the SAS are so skilled at hostage rescue that they are sometimes used in preference to American special forces when US citizens are taken hostage.

The good news ends there. Hostage situations are often fatal for the hostages. Even if the SAS do arrive, hostage rescue is such a dangerous process that innocents sometimes get killed. Hostages are often murdered during the negotiating stages of a hostage situation. And sometimes, of course, the authorities simply don't know where the hostages are being held.

These are not improbable scenarios. In November 2015, during the Bataclan theatre massacre in Paris, terrorists took a hundred innocent people hostage and threatened to decapitate one every five minutes. When armed police assaulted the venue, one of the terrorists exploded a suicide vest. The loss of life was horrific. In a Moscow theatre in 2002, Chechen rebels took civilians hostage, starting a two-and-a-half-day siege. It was only ended when Russian special forces filled the building with a chemical agent and raided it. The hostage-takers were killed, but so were more than one hundred hostages.

In this chapter, I want to explain to you how to increase your chances of staying safe at all stages of a hostage situation, from the initial abduction, through the process of being held, to the moment when – hopefully – a rescue team arrives. But be under no illusion: this is a life-threatening situation.

THE MOMENT OF ABDUCTION

A hostage-taker knows that this is the moment when their target has the greatest chance of thwarting an abduction. They are therefore just as likely to use guile as force.

A good example of this is a real-life abduction that took place in West London in a street where a very wealthy man lived. His house was well-protected with guards and up-to-date security systems. He was driving home one day, when a woman in another car crashed into him. An argument followed. The woman insisted that the crash was his fault and not hers. Irate, she called the police. A police car arrived. A policeman climbed out and examined the scene. The woman became very aggressive. The police officer told the man to go and sit in his police car while he dealt with the woman, telling him that she was going to get arrested. The man did as he was instructed.

The moment he sat in the back seat of the police car, two other men jumped into the front and sped off. The whole thing had been a set-up. They weren't real police officers. The guy had been abducted.

We're not finished with this story, but for now we need to

focus on one aspect of it: the length to which the abductors went to get the target into their vehicle. This is because abductions are hard, *if the target chooses to make them so.*

If you believe you are being abducted, you must do everything in your power to stop it happening. That means fighting. Be as violent as you can. Kick. Gouge. Bite. Scream. Fight like a lunatic. You have literally seconds to react. Even if they are armed, you need to ensure that your application of violence is intense and effective at this initial stage – your abductors probably don't want want a gunfight on the streets. If they overpower you, they'll get you into a vehicle and from there into a stronghold. Your chances of escape or rescue suddenly become much smaller. There's a good chance you'll never be seen again. Do what it takes to ensure that doesn't happen. Look at the chapter on fighting to gather some tips on effective counter-attacking techniques.

HOW TO BEHAVE WHILE YOU'RE BEING HELD

Maybe you haven't managed to avoid abduction. Whatever the specifics of your scenario, your behaviour probably needs to change if you're being held.

At this point, fighting, at least initially, is not your best course of action. How you behave will depend, of course, on your situation. Do you have one abductor or many? Are they armed? What are their aims? Are they demanding ransoms? Do they have explosives or even suicide belts?

If you think that your life is in immediate danger, you may need to fight if you possibly can. I can't make that call for you – it will be down to your assessment of the situation. In general, however, if you've been taken hostage your abductors will want you alive, at least for now. So you need to take the following into consideration.

Be the grey man (or woman)

When I was working with the Mexican *Federales*, they told me stories about kidnappings by the drug cartels. The cartels would regularly abduct the family members of wealthy businessmen, who would always pay the ransom the cartels demanded. Sometimes the businessmen would get the family members back. Other times, just for the hell of it, the cartels would chop their hostage's head off and mail it back to the family once they'd received the money.

If someone has taken you hostage, there is a very good chance that they're prepared to kill you. If you're one of a group of hostages and you're the one acting aggressively, noisily, being a pain, kicking off or bringing attention to yourself in any way, guess who they're going to nail first.

You need to make like an SAS operative and be the grey man. Hang your head. Be polite. Be quiet. Don't give your abductors any reason to single you out.

Observe

Just because you're being the grey man, it doesn't mean you're doing nothing. Far from it.

There was a famous prison break in America. Every day, when a prison warder came into his cell, the prisoner in question would examine the shape of his keys. Over time, he managed to memorise and replicate those keys to effect his escape. I have spoken to many prison officers, and they've all told me the same thing: you make a mistake if you imagine that these are dumb criminals. They are watching your every movement and every mannerism, trying to pick up on something they can use against you.

That is how you must be if you're taken hostage. Your brain and your powers of observation need to be working overtime. The more information you have about your abductors, the higher your chances of escape. How many of them are there? Are they armed? If so, how? What is their routine? Who are the leaders and who are the sheep? Who is the psychopath? Who is the fundamentalist and who is not so sure? Where are the entry and exit points where you're being held? What time is it? What clothes are your attackers wearing? Are their nails manicured? Are they wearing a wedding ring? If they're masked, would you be able to use these non-facial features to recognise them?

Your aim is to appear docile and a bit stupid, while simultaneously gathering as much intelligence as you can that might be of use to you over the following hours and days. The more information you gather, the greater your chance of escape, and the more you will be able to help out in a rescue attempt.

Make friends

Abductors try to dehumanise their hostages. If and when the time comes that they have to kill someone, it makes it easier if they don't think of them as real humans. You need an effective countermeasure to this behaviour. If you're allowed to talk, tell the hostages about your wife/husband and children (even if you don't have any). Try to find out what their interests are, and feign similar interests. Try to create bonds, because the more you do this, the more difficult they will find it to harm you.

Look for the weak link

I want to take you back to the kidnapping story about the wealthy man who was tricked into the fake police car. Having kidnapped him in broad daylight, his abductors took him to a barn in the home counties. It was here that the brains of the operation made his mistake. He hired a couple of dumb criminals to look after him. They allowed the wealthy man to start up a conversation with them. He asked what they were being paid and told them that, whatever it was, he'd give them double. Over a period of a few days he kept on at them, understanding that they weren't the sharpest tools in the box, and targeting their greed. The two idiots let him go, believing his promise to pay them. The wealthy man got back home and, acting on his information, the police arrested the whole mob.

Every group of people has its weak links. Identify the person who isn't as nasty as the others. The one who's willing to catch your eye and smile. The one who's willing to talk. That's who you need to build a rapport with. Flatter him. Get the prettiest girl in the hostage group to flutter her eyelashes at him. Tell him that, if it comes to it, you'll explain to the authorities that he looked after you well. Ingratiate yourself.

Identify escape routes

If a chance to escape presents itself, you should grab it. For this reason, you should be constantly on the lookout for escape routes. These will depend on the structure of the building where you're being held. In general, though, I would be looking for:

- Fire escapes – these are very difficult to lock from the inside, so they often present excellent escape routes
- Large air-conditioning ducts
- Laundry chutes in hotels or conference centres
- Service staircases

Never take your eye off the ball. There may be a moment when your abductors get sloppy and leave a door open, giving you the chance to run for it. (This is more likely if you haven't been giving them aggro – the more aggressive you are, the more they're going to watch you.)

Identify cover

This is particularly important if you see your abductors wearing suicide vests, or if it's clear that there are explosives on site. But it's important anyway, because as you'll read below, a hostage rescue is an explosive and dangerous moment. Look for furniture – desks you can hide under, sofas you can crouch behind – in the event of things going noisy. There may be shrapnel, rounds, flying debris. Look for places where you're potentially protected from all these.

Take advantage of the possibility that someone is listening

If the authorities are aware of your location, there is a good chance that surveillance personnel are listening in. Specialist teams may have made a covert approach on the stronghold to drill microphones and/or cameras through walls. There are even devices that can listen in to the conversation in a room from a distance by measuring the vibration of the window. You need to take tactical advantage of this. If you are allowed to speak, try to deliver intelligence that might be of use to a rescue team. Clearly you need to do this in such a way that you do not expose what you're up to. A good strategy is to deliver information in the form of a conversation with another hostage. 'I thought there were only five of them, but maybe there are seven ...'

The more information, however trivial, that you can supply to the rescue team, the higher their chances of a successful operation.

Beware of Stockholm syndrome

Stockholm syndrome — where hostages develop sympathy for their captors — is real. You need to guard against it. Be in no doubt: you are in the hands of violent criminals. They are probably prepared to kill you and may even be planning to do so. Don't feel sorry for them. Lie like your life depends on it, because it probably does. Befriend them if you can, but in the event of a rescue attempt, be prepared to point them out to your rescuers so they can be taken out.

UNDERSTANDING AND PREPARING FOR A HOSTAGE RESCUE SCENARIO

As mentioned above, if you are a UK citizen and you have been taken hostage anywhere in the world, any hostage rescue attempt *will* be carried out by the SAS.

There are three possible scenarios:

1. The abductors are in contact with the authorities and nego-
tiations are ongoing.
2. The abductors are not in contact with any authorities, and
are unaware that a rescue attempt is imminent.
3. The hostages' location is unknown and no rescue attempt is
imminent.

In scenario 1, the SAS are likely to deploy as soon as the abductors start killing hostages. But you need to be prepared for a
hostage rescue in scenarios 2 and 3, because you won't know
which scenario you are in.

Before I explain a standard SAS response to a hostage situation, there is something you need to understand. The Regiment
are brought in when there is no option other than the swift,
precise application of extreme violence. To illustrate this, and to
explain why it is so important to guard against Stockholm
syndrome, I want to tell you an inside story about the Iranian
Embassy siege – the hostage-rescue mission that brought the
SAS into the public eye for the first time.

The embassy siege was carried out by six armed terrorists. The
SAS entered once one of the twenty-six hostages had been
murdered. They killed five of the six hostage-takers. The remaining terrorist was a young guy and it may have been that a few of
the hostages felt some sympathy with him. Once the shooting
had stopped and the hostages were being evacuated, Regiment
members lined the stairs as the hostages exited. The young
guy was somehow bundled down the stairs, along with the
hostages and, for whatever reason, it was only when they exited
the building, where a reception team was grabbing everyone, that
he was identified as one of the terrorists.

He was grabbed by one of the younger SAS lads. Some of the older guys, who were lurking in the shadows of the building, called on the young Regiment trooper to push the terrorist back into the building. There was only one reason they wanted him to do that: so that they could dispense some quick, lethal Regiment justice.

The young trooper refused. He knew that the press had cameras all around. He was vilified by the old timers, but in truth he'd made the right call. If he had been seen pushing the terrorist back into the building to be shot, there's little doubt that there would have been a criminal investigation and the SAS, instead of being praised for their professionalism, would have had their reputations tarnished.

There are two things we need to learn from this. Firstly, anything that may appear like you are protecting a terrorist, because of Stockholm syndrome or for whatever reason, puts you in the line of fire. Secondly, when the SAS arrive, they are going to go out of their way to kill people. The shock and awe of a special-forces hostage rescue is horrifying. The noise, violence and confusion are off the scale. You need to make sure there is *no* chance that you will be mistaken for a hostage-taker.

How SAS hostage rescues work

I want to give you an idea of how an SAS hostage-rescue operation takes place. I'm not going to give you any secret operational detail, but I am going to give you enough to help you make some smart calls about your behaviour, if you should find yourself in this kind of scenario.

A hostage rescue will normally require the involvement of an entire squadron of thirty to forty men. They will be divided into a sniper team and an assault team. There will likely be support from 1 Para on the outer cordons, and from armed police if you're in the UK.

The sniper team will be in positions of cover. They might be ten metres from the stronghold where the hostages are being held, or they might be as much as 600 metres away. Either way, you won't know they're there. The snipers will be giving a running commentary of what they can see. This is listened to by the commander back in the command centre. If a sniper has a target in his sights, this will be noted in the command centre.

The assault team will prepare to enter the stronghold via every available entrance. This is so that they can dominate the attack, and ensure nobody escapes. They'll come in through windows, doors and might even have to breach a wall. They are very skilled at explosive methods of entry. They will probably be using shaped charges at each of the entry points, and they know how to work out the overpressures so that the shock waves of their explosives don't harm the hostages inside the building.

When the hostage rescue is green lit, the commander will know exactly how many hostage-takers the snipers have in their targets. On his word – 'Stand by, stand by . . . go!' – the snipers will take out their targets. Simultaneously, the doors and windows will be blown in and the assault team will make its multi-point entrance. They will likely use flashbangs, which will create smoke, noise and chaos, and excruciatingly painful CR gas. When they encounter hostage-takers, they will kill them. Their aim is to execute every hostage-taker in the building.

How you should prepare

First things first: you might be expecting the SAS to arrive, but whatever you do, keep quiet about it. Don't needle your captors that the Regiment are on their way. Don't even *mention* the SAS. The guys won't thank you for it. They want their arrival to be sudden and unexpected. They don't want the hostage-takers to take extra steps to prepare themselves for a hit, because you've made them think a bit harder about their own mortality.

You'll be wondering how long you've got to wait. You've no way of knowing. It could be an hour, it could be two or three days, or longer. But as soon as they start killing people, expect an assault.

If possible, keep away from doors and especially windows. Snipers will be firing through windows, and the assault teams will be blasting them in. That means you'll be in the vicinity of rounds, explosively shattering glass and doors flying in. If you can't move away from a window, position yourself below the ledge, and stay below it.

You should avoid interior walls, especially if they're hollow plasterboard stud walls – if there's any shooting (and there probably will be), rounds flying in adjoining rooms will rip easily through these. The best place to position yourself is against a solid exterior wall, but if possible, tuck yourself down in the corner. If the rescue team has to breach the wall, they'll probably do it in the centre where the structure is weaker.

Nothing can prepare you for the heart-stopping noise and sudden violence of a team coming in. It causes some people to freeze and numb up. You need to avoid this happening. The likelihood is that the team will have a list of all the hostages' names. Your aim is to make sure they know that you are a hostage and not a target. So: scream your name and your nationality. Keep your hands up where the guys can see them. If it's very smoky, which it probably will be, shout out your location. Keep shouting these pieces of information so that you are identifiable to the team.

There is a chance that the hostage-takers will dress you up to look like one of them. This might involve forcing you into a ski mask, taping or supergluing an unloaded weapon to your arm and making you walk around the stronghold. They're doing this to confuse any snipers and to make life more difficult for the assault team when it comes to identifying the correct targets. In fact, it's probably not going to confuse the snipers. If they're on the ground for long enough – maybe over a period of twenty-four hours – they'll soon observe that there's something unnatural about your movements. And the quality of their optics will mean that they'll probably be able to tell you have a weapon fixed to your hands. However, in the heat and confusion of a hostage rescue, there's still a danger of a mix-up. Get to the ground and lie on top of your weapon. As above, keep shouting out your name, nationality and position.

Don't expect to be treated gently. You may be plasticuffed and forced on to the ground. You'll probably be treated like a potential threat. Go with it. Do exactly what you're told. The men rescuing you will be ruthlessly professional, but they will be on a knife's edge. Don't give them any reason to make a mistake.

HOW TO DEAL WITH A TORTURE SITUATION

I've undergone tactical interrogation in training many times. It is psychologically and physically brutal. One thing is certain: you can't withstand it indefinitely. In the Regiment, you're expected to hold out for twenty-four hours, by which time any codes or frequencies that could be of use to an aggressor will have been changed, and the intel you'll ultimately end up spilling will be useless.

In a civilian scenario, if an aggressor is trying to get information from you by means of torture, give it to them immediately. There's nothing you can tell them that will harm national security. It's more likely to be personal information about bank accounts, safe combinations or the location of valuables. Hand it over.

It's possible, of course, that you're going to be tortured for sadistic reasons. If this happens, it will be terrible, but I would advise you not to fight it. The more you resist, the more aggressive your torturer is likely to become. Remember that you can't drown from waterboarding if it happens to you. Your only countermeasure is to try to relax and to give them any information they want. If you're being beaten with fists, bludgeons or rifle butts (and this is the most likely form of torture), I would advise you to let them hit your head. This is contrary to my usual advice about covering your head and neck in a conflict situation (see page 178 or 261), but in this instance, it can work to your advantage. Your head bleeds more profusely than the rest of your body. If your wounds *appear* dramatic, your aggressors are likely to lay off a little.

If you need to wet yourself or soil yourself, do it. It's humiliating, but if you're dirty and stinking, your aggressors will want to keep their distance. Let it go.

In the wake of the Bravo Two Zero mission, having escaped across Iraq and made it over the Syrian border, I found myself in the custody of two members of the Syrian secret police. They had their fun with me. They performed a mock execution, and made me believe that they were escorting me not to Damascus, but back to Baghdad: the one place in the world I was trying to avoid.

If I ended up in Baghdad, I'd be tortured. No question. I had to get my head in the right place. I started running over the probable sequence of events in my mind. I'm going to end up in an Iraqi military compound, I told myself. When I arrive there, they'll drag me out of the car. They'll immediately start beating me. They'll kick me, punch me and get me on the ground. Then they'll drag me into a building and start questioning me. They'll strip me naked. They'll humiliate me. If I refuse to answer their questions, they'll beat me round the head, torso and genitals . . .

Strange as it might sound, putting these scenarios into my head was an important survival mechanism. It meant that, if I did enter a torture situation, the actions of my aggressors wouldn't come as a shock. I knew I was in no physical state to fight these people, so I had to rely on my mental strength.

I am often asked if I have any psychological techniques for dealing with pain and fear. This is my advice: admit to yourself the possibility of what is about to happen. That way, you're not in for a double whammy of the event itself and the horrific shock of its occurrence.

CHRIS RYAN'S HOSTAGE SITUATION DEBRIEF

- In the moment of abduction, fight as dirtily, aggressively and noisily as you can. You have only seconds to stop this situation developing into something worse.
- Once you've been abducted, become the grey man. Don't attract attention to yourself, but be constantly vigilant and quietly gather as much information as you can.
- Stockholm syndrome is real. Remember: your abductors are criminals who will do you harm if necessary. They are your enemies, not your friends.
- In the event of a hostage rescue, shout your name, nationality and location so the team know who and where you are.
- Prepare yourself for torture situations by going through what might happen in your head. If it *does* happen, don't fight it. Give up any information you're asked for.

16

STAYING SAFE DURING A MASS TERROR INCIDENT

Terrorist atrocities are, sadly, an increasingly common occurrence in the UK. Although your chances of being caught up in one of these are small, I believe it would be foolish to discount it. It's in the very nature of these incidents that they target ordinary members of the public. Which means that ordinary members of the public need to be aware of the risks and to understand how they should react in the event of some of the more common types of attack. That's what I want to take you through in this chapter.

UNDERSTANDING TERROR THREAT LEVELS

Terror threat levels are established by the Joint Terrorism Analysis Centre. JTAC is based at MI5 headquarters. It analyses all available intelligence regarding terrorist threats, capabilities, intentions and timescales. The intelligence it has to work with is normally patchy. JTAC can only make judgements based on what it knows.

There are five different threat levels:

- Low: an attack is unlikely
- Moderate: an attack is possible, but not likely
- Substantial: there is a strong possibility of an attack
- Severe: there is a high likelihood of an attack
- Critical: an attack is expected at any time

The terror threat level for international terrorism (there is a separate threat level for Northern Ireland-related terrorism) has been available to the public since 2006. In that time, it has never been less than substantial. It moves to critical under exceptional circumstances, when security measures need to be moved to maximum in response to specific threats. As I write, it is severe. JTAC does not maintain this high threat level for no reason. That's why the information in this chapter is so important to you and your family.

FIREARMS-RELATED INCIDENTS

We have already discussed the Tunisian beach attacks on page 141. Sadly, firearms-related incidents are a possibility all over the world. They are commonplace in the US, of course, but events such as the Kenyan shopping-mall shootings, the Mumbai attacks, the *Charlie Hebdo* and Paris nightclub shootings, and the Dunblane school massacre are evidence that these are world-wide phenomena.

The standard police advice for a firearms attack is that you should *run* if you can run, *hide* if you can't and *tell* the authorities what's going on. I agree with this advice, but would like to expand on it based on my experience of being in firearms contact situations. To do this, I'm going to imagine you're in a shopping-mall-type firearms incident, or a nightclub shooting. You hear gunshot. What do you do?

Identifying gunfire

This can be more difficult than it sounds. As we saw with the Tunisian beach shootings, many holidaymakers made an initial assumption that the gunfire was somebody letting off fireworks.

Gunfire has a very distinctive crack and bang. If rounds are coming past you, you hear their passage and it sounds like the violent crack of a whip (take that as a signal that someone has a bead on you or you're in their line of sight). Rather than try to describe the sound of gunfire to you, however, I want to direct you to two movies where it is, in my opinion, absolutely realistic: *Saving Private Ryan* and *Heat*. *Heat* especially gives you a very accurate idea of the boom, cracks and echo of gunfire in an urban area.

Running

Evacuating yourself from the area should be your first response. You need to run. Leave all your belongings. Move quickly and quietly. Try to encourage others to come with you, but don't let them slow you down if they can't make their mind up.

It might sound obvious, but you need to be sure that you're running in the right direction. To do this, you must first use your eyes. Are people running *en masse*? If so, they're probably running away from the shooter. Can you see wounded or dead bodies? That's an indication that you're running toward the shooter.

However, you can't *rely* on your eyes. People might be running randomly. They may be being herded into an ambush. There may be no bodies. That's where your hearing comes in. If there is gunfire, listen to it. This is particularly important in a shopping mall, where networks of corridors hit each other at right angles and cause the noise to echo. The closer you are to the source of the gunfire, the louder, sharper and more distinct it will be. If you're further away, of course, it will be less distinct and echo more.

You need to think calmly and carefully about your exits. The main exits to a building may not be your best bet. In a shopping mall, for example, it's worth remembering that every individual shop has a loading bay or fire exit at the back. That's where I would head – especially if it became apparent that the main exits were blocked off. I would encourage other people to come with me – there is safety in numbers – and I would get a shop attendant to join us, not only for their own safety, but also because they'll have access cards or keypad codes to the restricted areas behind the shop.

If you're in sight of the gunman and are running away from him, say down a mall corridor, you should move in a zigzag. This means you present a laterally moving target, which is more difficult to hit. Tuck your head down to make yourself a smaller target.

If you're in a more enclosed space, such as a music venue or nightclub, there will be mass panic and low lighting. The threat of being crushed or suffocated in a stampede is almost as great as the threat from a shooter, so it is essential that you do everything you can to stay on your feet. The temptation might be to get on the ground, but if you do that, you risk death by trampling.

In such a scenario, I would be thinking to myself: where did the shooter or shooters enter? The most likely entrance point is the easiest: the main entrance. So, to get away from the shooter, you would need to get toward the stage area where the artists come in, or toward a fire escape. Try to get to the edge of the room and work your way along the walls – you will probably come to an exit. If not, keep forcing yourself toward the rear of the building, where there undoubtedly *will* be an exit. If you are following a wall to find an exit, keep about a foot away from it – this means that you're out of range of a ricocheting round.

These two scenarios assume that you are on the ground floor of a building. This may not be the case. If you find yourself on the first floor and can smash through a window, you may be able to escape that way. Don't try to do a movie star running jump, however. Find a window with an outdoor ledge. Clamber out and hang from the ledge – this reduces the height of your fall. Make sure you don't lock your legs when you hit the ground – keep them slightly bent and roll to one side on impact, like a parachute landing. And of course, be very vigilant that you're not falling on to dangerous ground, or into a basement. Be aware that you risk breaking an ankle or even a leg if you do this: you have to make a decision about whether this is a risk worth taking.

If you're higher than the first floor, don't try to jump. You'll need to make an assessment about whether you should run, based on what you know about the shooter's location and movements. It may be that your safest option is to hide.

Once you've exited the area of a firearms incident, don't assume you're safe. In our shopping-mall scenario, it's very possible that the shooters will spill out into the loading bays behind the shops. In a music venue or nightclub, they may well move to the backstage area. If the gunman is still at large, never let your guard down. Continue moving away from the area. If you can't do that, find a place to hide.

And in general, if you can't move to safety via a route that will not put you in the line of fire, you should hide.

Hiding

See pages 201–4 for more detail on how to hide and why things are seen. Here I want to give you some more specific advice for hiding during a firearms incident.

If someone has a weapon, you need a substantial physical barrier between you and them. Try to find a place with thick, reinforced walls – rounds can easily pass through plasterboard stud walls. Try to avoid dead ends and bottlenecks. It can be a good idea to lock yourself inside a room. If you do this, remember that the door is probably a weak point through which rounds can pass, especially if it's a wooden interior door. Stay away from it.

So: if you're in a shopping mall, a locked store room is a better hiding place than crouching behind a till, which will only ever be a temporary point of cover. In a nightclub, there'll be a lockable admin office or a dressing room. If you can't lock yourself into these rooms, barricade them from the inside with heavy items of furniture, which will also mitigate against bullet penetration.

Once you've hidden, keep absolutely silent. Don't shout for help. Turn off your phone and make sure it's not set to vibrate, because this still makes a noise that will identify your position.

If you've hidden in an enclosed space, do not move. Stay hidden, even when things have gone quiet. Only reveal yourself when you're absolutely certain that the police have arrived and the shooter is neutralised.

Contacting the police

If you can do so without drawing attention to yourself, call 999 or the appropriate emergency number for the country you're in. Don't assume somebody else has done it. They may be panicking. They may be dead.

You need to give the police as much intel as possible, such as:

- Your location.
- A description of the attackers.
- Whether there are any casualties.
- Access and exit points if you're in a building.
- A description of the shooter's weapons (see pages 211–19 for more on this).
- Anything you know about the shooter's location.

You may be asked to keep the line open, so that you can maintain contact with the police. When they arrive, they will be armed. Expect them to be abrupt, even rough. Remember that they may not be sure whether you're a gunman or an innocent bystander. Make no sudden movements, keep your hands visible at all times, try to keep calm and do *everything* they tell you to do.

What to do when you're cornered by a gunman

Sometimes you can't run. Sometimes you can't hide. There is a gunman in the vicinity. You're cornered. What now?

In a scenario such as a shopping-mall or nightclub shooting, you can be fairly sure that the gunman won't be experienced or very highly trained. You need to get to a point of cover and watch them like a hawk, because at some point – especially if they are using a semi-automatic pistol, a submachine gun or an assault rifle, and as you will understand if you have read the chapter on what you need to know about firearms – there is a chance of a stoppage. There's an even bigger chance that they'll run out of ammunition.

An SAS man is trained to count his rounds. It's hard-wired. To this day, if I'm watching a movie and I see a character with a revolver (six rounds) or an automatic pistol (twelve rounds), I'll be counting each round as it's discharged. It's amazing how often they have more rounds than they do in real life. In a contact situation, I'll be counting my own rounds and my enemy's. If they've got a Kalashnikov assault rifle with thirty rounds and they're firing in bursts of three or four rounds on automatic, I'll know they have nine or ten bursts, depending on how disciplined they are.

In a firearms-related terror incident, it may be difficult to keep tabs on this. But the chances are the same will be true of the shooter. They'll be shooting, and suddenly no more rounds will be coming from their weapon. You'll see them look at it momentarily. Then you'll see them putting their hand underneath the weapon to remove the magazine.

That's your chance.

You have a window of opportunity to overpower the gunman when they're changing their magazine. Move fast and be brutal. You have just seconds to put him down. See pages 177–84 for how to make sure your attack is effective.

Clearly, attacking an armed man is a last resort, only to be considered if you can't run or hide.

VEHICLE-RAMMING INCIDENTS

Vehicle-ramming attacks – such as those performed on Westminster Bridge and London Bridge in 2017 – are not new, but they are increasingly common. This is because the only weapon needed is a vehicle, and these are easy to come by. If somebody has it in their head to commit such an atrocity, there is very little the authorities can do about it.

Before we discuss our best responses to such an incident, I want to give a snapshot of exactly what happened during the Westminster Bridge and London Bridge incidents.

At approximately 14.40 on 22 March 2017, Khalid Masood mounted the pavement heading south over Westminster Bridge. He drove along the pavement at a speed of more than seventy miles per hour, hitting pedestrians and forcing one woman to jump over the side of the bridge. Thirty seconds later, he hit the perimeter fence of the Palace of Westminster.

He left the vehicle and, armed with a knife, ran toward the Houses of Parliament. Here he stabbed and killed an armed police officer, Keith Palmer, before being shot by armed officers. The attack lasted eighty-two seconds, injured fifty and killed five.

At approximately 22.00 on 3 June 2017, a van containing three terrorists mounted the pavement at the northern end of London Bridge. It swerved on and off the pavement at a speed of about fifty miles per hour, hitting pedestrians. One of the pedestrians was knocked into the river and his body was later found downstream. On the south side of the bridge it crashed into a pub. The three men emerged, armed with ceramic knives. They were wearing fake suicide vests. They ran toward nearby Borough Market, slashing and stabbing people as they went. As they moved through Borough Market, members of the public started throwing crates, chairs and glasses at them. They still managed to stab one of their victims between ten and fifteen times. At 22.16, armed police arrived. They shot and killed the three attackers. A member of the public was also shot. Forty-eight people were injured. Eight were killed.

From the point of view of the terrorist, bridges are particularly effective locations to carry out a vehicle ramming, because the escape routes of the pedestrians he is trying to hit are limited. And cities are good because there are plenty of targets, most of whom are habitually unaware of their surroundings. They don't know they're under attack until the vehicle hits them, and by then it's too late.

Your response to a vehicle-ramming incident can only ever be reactive. For this reason, your best defence against such an attack is – as always – heightened situational awareness. If you're walking across Westminster Bridge with your earphones in while reading messages on your phone, you've taken your two most important senses – sight and hearing – out of the equation. If a vehicle is hurtling toward your back, your warning sign will be the reaction of oncoming pedestrians and the sound of shouting and screaming. In the chapter on staying safe in the street, I advised you always to be hyper-alert to your environment. In a world where terrorists drive vehicles into crowds of innocent pedestrians, this is even more important. Remember our colour-code system. Maintain Condition Yellow. Be alert for the sight of speeding vehicles and the sound of revving engines.

When you're walking along the pavement, try to face oncoming traffic. This may give you the few seconds' warning you need.

Many roads have bollards separating the pavement from the road itself, in order to deter this kind of attack. I would always choose these routes if possible.

If you're involved in a vehicle-ramming incident, your escape routes will depend entirely on the scenario. If you can see the vehicle approaching, try to assess its speed and how many seconds you have to make an evasive manoeuvre. If possible, run in the direction from which the attack vehicle drove. This will, of course, mean running past the vehicle, so you'll need to make an in-the-moment assessment of whether this is sensible. You will probably have to get on to the road itself, so be wary of other road users before you do this. Especially, be very aware that there may be a follow-up vehicle ready to ram those who are escaping.

If the incident occurs on a bridge, and you can't get behind the vehicle, and your assessment is that it's too close and moving too fast for you to run away, it may be that your only escape route is into the water. This is extremely high-risk. One woman was forced to do this during the Westminster Bridge attack. She survived, but her injuries were serious. In this situation, suddenly the biggest threat to your life isn't the terrorist, but the river. Remember that people commit suicide by jumping off bridges, and they mostly die from the impact of hitting water. Even if you survive that impact, you might be knocked unconscious, or break bones that will make swimming impossible. It will be cold – the temperature change can cause cold-water shock, which can lead to hyperventilation and even heart attack. The gasp response may cause you to inhale water. This happened to a friend of mine who tried to help someone who'd lost control of their canoe. He jumped into the water, which was so cold that it caused him to empty his lungs and then suck in the water. He was dead in less than a minute.

So, if you have no option other than to jump off a bridge, here's what to do. Look down. Make an assessment of what is below you. Is there any river debris that you need to avoid (unlikely in a city river)? Are you going to land against the uprights of the bridge? If you're wearing a winter coat or any heavy clothing, get rid of it, because it'll drag you down. Take a deep breath. Prepare yourself for the fact that it's going to be cold: keep your mouth shut and concentrate on keeping it shut. Step off the bridge. Stay upright with your hands by your side and your legs slightly bent – this will reduce the impact of the water, but it will still be substantial, so prepare yourself for that. When you hit the water, put all your effort into keeping your mouth shut. You'll sink, but then you should naturally rise to the surface. When you do, you need to make an assessment of the direction of the current. Don't fight it – you'll exhaust yourself and drown. Instead, you need to look downstream and fix a point on the shore toward which you can swim at a forty-five-degree angle, while the current moves you in that direction.

I hope I've persuaded you that jumping off a bridge is a last resort. I would always try to choose other escape routes, if possible. Grab your chance when you can. If the vehicle has hit something or someone, grab the opportunity to get away. If you can find immediate cover to protect you from the impact of a vehicle, you can consider that. But remember that the force of a speeding vehicle is substantial. Getting behind a lamppost, for example, might afford you some protection if you have no other option, but you're still likely to be severely wounded if the vehicle hits it.

Remember that in both the Westminster Bridge and the London Bridge incidents, the vehicle-ramming itself has been followed up with serious, fatal knifing incidents. Just because the vehicle has stopped, it doesn't mean the threat has passed. It's probably just beginning. Escaping the immediate vicinity of the vehicle is not enough. Keep running and try to get indoors, but bear in mind the following advice about knife attacks.

KNIFE ATTACKS

No right-thinking person could have been anything other than horrified by the sickening attack on Fusilier Lee Rigby near the Royal Artillery Barracks in London. The young soldier was hit by a vehicle, stabbed with knives and hacked with a meat cleaver. Once he was dead, his killers attempted to decapitate him before shooting and wounding two members of the armed police-response unit.

Terrorists like knives and other blades because they are easily acquired, unlike firearms (at least in the UK), and they're very easy to conceal. A knife attacker never runs out of ammunition, a good knife will cut through pretty much anything, and it's easy for an assailant to target his or her victim's most vulnerable points with a knife. For these reasons, they are more of a threat to civilians than firearms are.

These types of attack are on the up, as we know from the events after the Westminster Bridge and London Bridge attacks described above. I want to give you some tips on what your response to such an incident should be.

Distance

A knife is a contact weapon. If a knife attacker can't get close to you, he can't hurt you. All the usual advice about moving away from the field of conflict applies, but in a knife attack situation you can use quite small distances to your advantage. If you can set an object – a parked car, for example, or a heavy table – between you and the attacker, you can keep circling and maintain the crucial distance between yourself and the contact weapon. In doing this, you buy yourself time, either for the police to arrive, or to identify incidental weapons, or to marshal a crowd response, as I will explain below.

The worst thing you can do is to turn your back on someone wielding a knife close by, or to hunker down and clam up.

You can do nothing to defend yourself in either of these positions – you simply give your aggressor the opportunity to stab you.

Find weapons

If you're cornered by one or more aggressors wielding knives and there's no escape route, you have to move into attack mode. You must look for weapons. This might mean grabbing a chair or smashing a bottle, so you have a weapon with which to glass the aggressor. Liquids – hot or cold – are very good tools for momentarily suppressing an attacker. A fire extinguisher will hold them back and keep the crucial distance between you.

Encourage other people to fight with you, and use projectiles. If you have lots of people throwing lots of objects at the attackers, it will help you to dominate them. This was the natural response of the crowd and security guards when the London Bridge attackers went marauding through the bars of Borough Market with knives. The crowds threw bottles, pint glasses and chairs at the attackers: a response that I'm certain will have saved lives.

Overcoming a knife man with hand-to-hand combat

If it's just you and him, there's a high chance that you're going to get slashed or stabbed. There are certain areas of your body where you really don't want this to happen, namely your major arteries, major veins and vital organs. In practice, this means protecting your torso, throat and the insides of your arms and legs. In particular, be aware of and protect the line down the centre of your body: this core line covers your throat, heart, lungs and many arteries. We only have to see what happened to the brave police officer Keith Palmer, who was killed with a knife outside Parliament during the Westminster Bridge attack, to understand how devastating these wounds can be. He was wearing a protective vest, but that's often not enough protection against a sharp knife to the body.

It's much better – though obviously still dangerous – to present the front of your forearms as you go in to attack. If you have time, you should wrap them with protective material. This might be an article of clothing or a belt – anything to give your arms a bit of protection against the knife (and to act as a bandage if you do get slashed).

You need to focus on their weapon arm rather than the weapon itself. This can be difficult, because you'll be worried about the blade slicing you. But it's the arm you need to control, not the blade. If you control the arm, you control the person. When people are wielding a knife, they tend to forget that they can use their other limbs against you. Disable the arm – sit on it, break it, do whatever you have to do – and you disable their ability to harm you, at least temporarily.

The best way to dominate a knife man completely is to encourage a group of people to overcome him. It needs to be a coordinated attack. One person goes for the knife arm. Others go for the remaining limbs. Once you have him on the ground, you don't hold back. Remember: he wants to kill you. Use the knife on him if you can wrest it from his grip. Otherwise, attack his face. Gouge his eyes if you have to. Stab him with pens, hit him with incidental weapons. Completely overpower him with relentless and effective violence, but *do not free his knife arm while he is still holding his weapon.*

BOMBS AND IEDS

Modern bombs and IEDs (improvised explosive devices) are sophisticated and devastating. A relatively small device can cause damage over a surprisingly wide area. An IED with 3kg of high explosive will easily take out an entire floor of a large office building. A military Claymore will take out a football pitch.

The big problem is that military-grade explosives are not that hard to come by on the black market. It is scraped out of unexploded munitions in former war zones. Add some improvised shrapnel – coins, or nuts and bolts that you can buy in any DIY store – plus a rudimentary detonator, and you have an extremely deadly device.

The additional problem we have to contend with is that terrorists are becoming increasingly skilled at disguising IEDs as ordinary objects. At the height of the conflict in Afghanistan, Taliban fighters were able to make their devices practically indistinguishable from rocks. In an urban environment, it's even easier. Devices can be hidden in bins, vehicles, suitcases, or pretty much any other object that you might see in the street.

This is why, as always, we must be hyper-aware of our surroundings. It is important to be suspicious of anything that seems remotely out of place. Don't ignore those signs and warnings to be careful of unattended bags. If you see someone placing an object in a public place – a workman placing a bin on a railway station concourse, for example – don't assume that they're doing so in an official capacity. Terrorists don't act in the shadows when they want to plant a device in a crowded area. They do it in plain sight, when they know most members of the public are too busy or switched off to notice them.

Having served in Northern Ireland during the Troubles, I remain particularly vigilant about car suspension. If I see a parked vehicle with no passengers, but which is low down on its suspension, I know there's something heavy in the boot. It might only be luggage, but it might be something more sinister. I would definitely avoid that vehicle. (When the IRA planted car bombs, they used to jack up the suspension to mitigate against this warning sign.)

The uncomfortable truth is that if you fail to notice an IED, there's little you can do to avoid the horrific effects of its blast. Your safety, and that of your family, depends on circumstance.

However, if you survive the initial blast, you need to think tactically, because the incident may not be over yet.

My brother served with the Parachute Regiment in Afghanistan. He told me a story about a patrol that was travelling up a valley in Helmand Province, when it had a contact with a group of four Taliban fighters. They reacted according to standard operating procedures: each man found cover before laying down fire. Some of the guys ran to the base of a tree, some into a hollow in the ground, some to a wall. They killed the insurgents and went on their way.

What they didn't realise, however, was that they were being watched by some tribal elders. These elders noted the exact positions the patrol members had chosen for cover.

Six months later, another patrol was travelling the same route. They got into a contact with another team of insurgents, and sought cover in exactly the same locations. This is what the Taliban knew they would do. They had planted IEDs in those places. The patrol was wiped out.

If I survived a bombing – or indeed any other mass terror incident – my immediate thoughts would be: where do the terrorists expect me to run, and where might they have hidden a secondary device? I would avoid running in the obvious direction with the crowd, and I would be on extra high alert for rubbish bins, vehicles or suspicious packages of any kind. My priority would be to get to open ground, where there is less likelihood of a hidden device.

SUICIDE BOMBERS

There was a time when suicide bombers were a threat restricted to the war zones of the Middle East. No longer. On 22 May 2017, a suicide bomber detonated a homemade shrapnel bomb at an Ariana Grande concert in Manchester Arena, killing twenty-three adults and children and injuring more than a hundred others. We need to get used to the idea of suicide bombs as a fact of modern life.

Suicide bombings are probably the most difficult type of mass terror incident to mitigate against. If armed police or the SAS are on to a suicide bomber, their strategy will be to take him out with a head shot, but even this is a risk: the bomber may be holding a pressure release detonator. As soon as he releases it, which would happen in the event of his death, the suicide vest explodes.

A civilian's only real defence against a suicide bomber is to identify them before they have a chance to detonate. So, as always, situational awareness, especially in crowded, confined areas, is essential. You need to be constantly aware of the people around you. It's your only way of anticipating an attack.

Statistically, a suicide bomber is most likely to be male and between the ages of seventeen and thirty-five. They are very likely to be political or religious extremists.

A suicide bomber's clothing will probably look out of place and unseasonal. They will almost certainly have a jacket on, and it will make them look unnaturally bulky, almost as though they're wearing body armour. Either that, or the clothing will look very baggy.

Alternatively, the suicide bomb will be in a backpack. If this is the case, they may be gripping it very firmly. They will certainly be being very careful with it. During the July 7th suicide-bomb attack on London, one of the targets was a London bus. A survivor of the attack remembered how the bomber was very careful not to let his backpack brush against her as he entered the bus while she was talking to the driver. She thought it meant he was being polite. Far from it. People are generally not that careful about their backpacks. If they're taking special care, be wary.

A suicide bomber is likely to loiter while they try to locate the best position to detonate. This means they will be moving differently to the general thrust of the crowd. If they are walking, they are likely to walk slowly. This helps them with surveillance – they can tell more easily if someone is approaching them at speed.

The detonating switch will often be taped to the bomber's hand, which means that he will want to keep it in his pocket. However, it may be on another part of his body. This may lead him nervously and repeatedly to touch the area of clothing where the switch is concealed.

Not all suicide bombers are of Muslim origin, but if they are, it is common for them to shave all their body hair as part of a pre-martyrdom ritual. So, if there is lighter skin tone on the beard area, or evidence below the neck that body hair has been shaved, this is another potential indicator.

A suicide bomber will mostly look nervous. They may be sweating. They may be looking anxiously around. They may be muttering a prayer to themselves.

None of these characteristics are definite indicators of a suicide bomber, of course. But if you see clusters of them, you need to take steps.

If you suspect a suicide bomber, it's very important that you don't call him out. This will cause mass panic, and will most likely force the bomber into detonating. Your only effective response as a civilian is to move yourself and your family quickly and quietly away from the area. If you're in an enclosed area such as a music venue, get to the exit or, at the very least, to another room so that the walls can act as a ballistic shield between you and the bomb. Only then should you raise the alarm. Call 999, or try to find a police officer. If the police officer is armed, so much the better, but be aware that no police officer is going to use a firearm against a member of the public merely because you say they're wearing a big coat and you can't see their hands.

If you can't get away, and you believe a suicide attempt is imminent, you have a choice to make.

Choice one: find cover, as solid and as large as possible. When a suicide vest filled with shrapnel goes off, it's going to spread randomly over a very wide area. If you don't have cover, you're highly likely to take some of it. If there's no cover, get on to the ground in a foetal position, with your hands covering your head and neck. This protects your vital organs. You may still take shrapnel, but you'll have a better chance of survival.

Choice two: look at the bomber's hands. If you can see them, try to identify if he is holding a detonator. If you are sure that he *isn't*, you have a chance to overpower him by controlling his hands so that he cannot reach the detonating switch. But this is an extremely high-risk option, because there may be a remote detonator, operated by a third party.

And sadly, the only other piece of advice I can give you with respect to such incidents is that you can fight suicide with suicide. If you are able to wrestle a suicide bomber to the ground and cover him with your own body, you'll absorb much of the blast when the bomb goes off. You'll be killed, of course, and there will likely still be casualties, but they will be fewer. Whether you're prepared to be the hero of the day is something only you can decide, but if *my* daughter was in the kill zone, I know what I would do . . .

CHRIS RYAN'S MASS TERROR INCIDENT DEBRIEF

- Learn to identify the sound of gunfire.
- Run. Hide. Contact the police.
- If you're cornered by a gunman, watch for the moment that he has a stoppage.

- Heightened situational awareness is your best defence against a vehicle-ramming incident.
- Keep your distance from a knife man. Identify incidental weapons. Protect your vital organs and major veins and arteries.
- Learn how to identify a suicide bomber. Get away.

17

POST-TERROR INCIDENT FIRST AID

All Regiment soldiers are well versed in emergency medical procedures, and every SAS patrol will have a specialist medic among them. Some of the techniques we learn for saving lives on the battlefield will be of direct use in the wake of a terror attack. It is likely that there will be a high number of casualties after such an incident. They might be members of your family, and their injuries will probably be life-threatening. Knowing how to respond to these injuries in the minutes between a terror attack and the arrival of the emergency services can mean the difference between life and death. I want to share that information with you in this chapter.

CONSIDER YOUR OWN SAFETY

This is important. You do nobody any favours if you put yourself at risk. If you're hurt because you've not been mindful of your own safety, it means firstly that you can't help anybody else and secondly that you make the situation worse for the first responders.

The moments after a terror attack will be confusing, unpleasant and frightening. Try to see through that. Maintain your situational awareness and be constantly vigilant for further threats.

CALL FOR HELP

Again, don't assume someone else has done it. Any first aid you are able to give in such an incident is only ever going to be temporary. Many casualties will need emergency interventions and specialist medical care that you can't provide. Make sure it's on its way as a matter of priority.

FOCUS ON THE QUIET ONES

If somebody is screaming in pain, it's a good sign, relatively speaking. It means they're conscious, and breathing. They might be in agony, but your priority in the wake of a terror incident isn't pain relief, it's survival. You need to focus on the casualties who *aren't* screaming, because they're unconscious and/or not breathing. They're the ones who require immediate attention.

People with broken bones make a lot of noise, but this is seldom a life-threatening injury.

FOCUS ON THE CHILDREN

This is not sentimental, it's medical. Children have less blood in their body and can bleed out much more quickly. Their lungs are smaller, so lung damage is more catastrophic. If you have to make the choice between treating a child or an adult, treat the child first.

UNCONSCIOUS CASUALTIES

If a casualty is unconscious, your immediate priority is to check that their airway is open and that they are breathing. To do this:

- Put one hand on their forehead and tilt the head back.
- Put the index and middle finger of your other hand under their chin. Lift it slightly.
- Put your ear next to their mouth and listen for breathing. See if you can feel breath on your cheek.
- Look at their chest to see if it is rising. If it's not, don't wait any longer than ten seconds.

If the casualty is breathing

Put them in the recovery position, if it is safe to do so. To do this:

- With the casualty lying on their back, kneel next to them.
- Place the arm nearest you at a right-angle position, with the hand pointing upward.
- Tuck the other hand under their head, so the back of their hand is touching their cheek.
- Bend the knee that is furthest from you at a right angle.
- Gently roll the casualty on to their side.
- Check their airway again by tilting back their head and gently lifting their chin.
- Monitor them until help arrives.

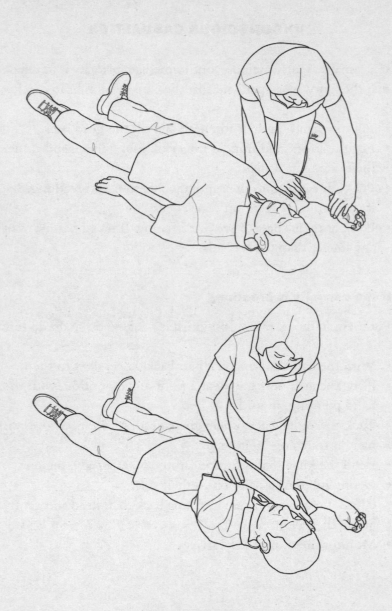

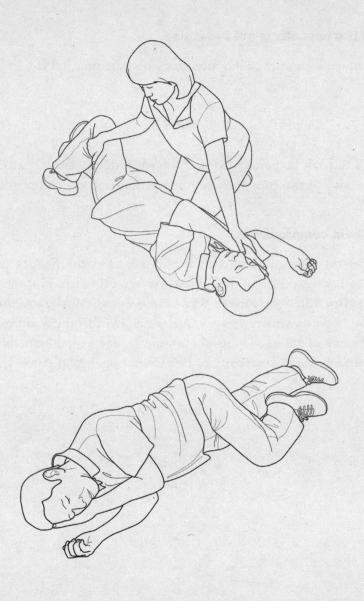

If the casualty is not breathing

Immediately start cardiopulmonary resuscitation (CPR).

CPR

CPR must be performed on a non-breathing casualty only. It consists of two phases: chest compressions and rescue breaths.

Chest compressions

Get on your knees next to the casualty. Put the heel of one hand at the centre of their chest. Put the other hand on top of the first. Interlock your fingers. Lean over the casualty and press the chest down five to six centimetres. Do this thirty times at the rate of 100–120 beats per minute. (Some people remember this as being the pulse of the Bee Gees song 'Stayin' Alive'.)

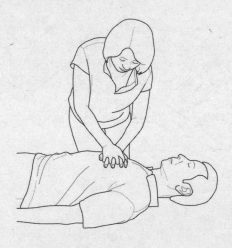

Rescue breaths

Pinch the casualty's nose. Open their mouth. Place your mouth over the casualty's, making sure that it's sealed tight. Blow into their mouth until their chest rises. Repeat.

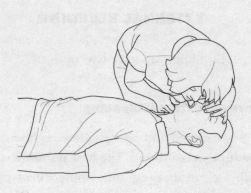

This sequence of thirty chest compressions followed by two rescue breaths must be alternated, until the casualty starts to breathe normally, or help arrives. If they start to breathe normally, put them in the recovery position as above.

CPR in children

The CPR process is slightly different for children.

If they are over one year old, start with five rescue breaths. Now continue with the cycle of thirty chest compressions and two rescue breaths as above. Make sure the chest is compressed by five centimetres.

If they are under a year old, the sequence is the same as for older children, but you apply the chest compressions more lightly: place two fingers in the middle of the chest, and compress by one third of its depth. (Only use the heel of your hand if you can't achieve that depth with your fingers.)

EXTERNAL BLEEDING

If a casualty is bleeding, you have two options.

Straightforward external bleeding

If the blood is dark red and not fast-flowing, the casualty has a straightforward external bleed. The best response is to pack the wound with a clean dressing, then apply direct pressure to it, through the dressing, for at least ten minutes. Of course, in the wake of a terror incident, you probably won't have a clean dressing, so you'll have to improvise with a T-shirt or any other piece of absorbent material. Don't be squeamish – get it right into the wound and apply strong pressure.

If there is an object, such as a piece of shrapnel, embedded in the wound, pad and apply direct pressure on either side of the object rather than directly on to it.

Catastrophic external bleeding

Sometimes, a casualty will be bleeding out so fast that they are likely to die in a minute or two. This normally happens when an artery has been cut. You can recognise an arterial bleed, because the blood will be very bright red and flowing very fast. This often, but not always, happens when a limb has been fully or partially amputated. In an instance like this, direct pressure may not work. We need to take a leaf out of the book of soldiers in Iraq and Afghanistan and make use of a tourniquet.

Be aware that tourniquets are not part of standard first-aid procedure. If you use them incorrectly, they can make blood-loss worse and ultimately cause casualties to lose limbs. You should only use them if bleeding is genuinely catastrophic and direct pressure is not working or impossible.

In essence, a tourniquet is a strap that is applied at least five centimetres above the wound. It is then tightened *extremely* tightly until the bleeding stops being life-threatening. You can buy combat application tourniquets commercially. I'd recommend keeping them in a domestic, office or vehicle's first-aid kit (with the proviso that they are never used unless absolutely necessary). These tourniquets have a windlass – a stick that you twist to get the strap really tight – and a label for recording the time the tourniquet is applied, which is important information for the medics.

In the wake of a terrorist event, you may have to improvise using a belt or any other material that can act as a strap – it should be at least an inch and a half in width to work properly. You'll know it's tight enough if your casualty shouts with pain.

SHRAPNEL WOUNDS

If a casualty has been in the vicinity of a suicide bomb or IED, there is a good chance that they will have pieces of shrapnel embedded in their body. This will cause bleeding. Treat the bleed as above, and perform CPR if necessary, but don't try to remove the shrapnel. There's a chance that it will be blocking a major artery. If this is the case, removing it will cause a catastrophic bleed.

GUNSHOT WOUNDS

Gunshot wounds can cause massive internal bleeding, fractured bones and major organ damage. You won't be in a position to treat any of these. But you will be in a position to deal with the external bleeding until the medics get on the scene.

It's very important to remember that firearm rounds can cause an entry wound *and* an exit wound, and sometimes more than one of each. One of the lads in the Regiment was shot in the ankle during the first Gulf War. The round passed through his leg, exited from his calf, re-entered his thigh and exited again at his backside. Thankfully he was worked on by a very skilled Iraqi surgeon and survived (although he did have a bit of a limp for while!) The lesson, however, is that you need to investigate the whole area of a gunshot wound and deal with all entry and exit wounds as above: pack the wounds with a T-shirt or dressing and keep direct pressure on them. If the casualty becomes unresponsive, check his or her airway and perform CPR if necessary.

KNIFE WOUNDS

Knife wounds can cause straightforward or catastrophic bleeding, and should be treated as above. If a knife has caused an abdominal wound, you should lie the casualty on their back and get them to bring their knees up – this closes the abdominal muscles. Place a large dressing or T-shirt over the wound.

BURNS

Explosive devices can cause serious burns. There are different degrees of burn, and a casualty's response to them is not always a good indicator of how serious they are – very bad burns can be less painful, because they destroy the nerve endings.

If possible, burns should be flooded with cool water. Remove any clothing or jewellery near to the burn, unless it is stuck to the skin, in which case leave it.

If necessary, treat the casualty for shock.

SHOCK

Shock is a medical condition – distinct from 'emotional' shock – that often follows, among other things, a severe bleeding injury or burn. It occurs when the circulatory system fails to deliver sufficient oxygen to the body's vital organs. It can result in death. Symptoms of shock include:

- pale, clammy or blue-tinged skin

- slow return of colour to the skin when a fingernail or toenail is pressed
- dizziness and/or nausea
- feeling cold
- fast, shallow breathing
- restless or aggressive behaviour
- confusion
- tiredness
- lack of consciousness

If you suspect shock, you need to monitor the casualty until the medics arrive. Lie them on their back and raise their legs above the level of their heart. Rest the legs on an object to keep them raised, or get someone to hold them up if necessary. Cover the casualty with a blanket or coat to keep them warm, and give them constant reassurance. If they lose consciousness, be prepared to get them into the recovery position or to administer CPR if necessary.

CRUSH INJURIES

These might occur in a vehicle-ramming incident or if heavy objects have fallen on a casualty during a bombing incident. In general, if you can remove someone from a crush situation, do so – *unless* they've been crushed for more than fifteen minutes, in which case you should leave them where they are. If possible, treat bleeding as above. If they are unconscious and not breathing, administer CPR – in position, if necessary and possible.

If you suspect a head injury, even a minor one, the casualty must be constantly monitored – especially if they seem confused. Head injuries can deteriorate badly. Be prepared to administer CPR if they become unconscious.

If you suspect a spinal injury, the casualty should not be moved – the slightest movement, especially of the head, can cause major damage.

CHRIS RYAN'S POST-TERROR INCIDENT FIRST-AID DEBRIEF

- Be mindful of your own safety. If you compromise that, you can't help others.
- Call for help. The casualties will need professional medics. Anything you do can only be a stop-gap.
- Casualties screaming in pain are lower priority than silent casualties.
- Learn CPR. It's different for adults and children.
- External bleeding: pack wounds and apply pressure. Tourniquets only for catastrophic, uncontrolled bleeding.
- Know the signs of shock. It can kill.

18

STAYING SAFE DURING A BIOCHEMICAL OR NUCLEAR ATTACK

When I was a young SAS soldier, the Cold War was still being waged. The Western powers knew that there was a threat of conventional, biological, chemical or even nuclear attack from the East. One of the potential battle fronts was the border between West Germany and East Germany. If the Russians attacked, there was a good chance that they would attack from this line. As a result, I was deployed there on a regular basis.

One of the Regiment's jobs along the German border was to dig in MEXE shelters. These are metal-framed tents covered with a sturdy, protective tarpaulin, about seven feet long and five feet wide. Enough room for a four-man patrol. Just. We would dig deep holes in the ground, big enough to bury the shelters, which would then be covered with a good eighteen inches of earth. We'd mark their location on a map, before checking the condition of previously installed shelters.

The purpose of these MEXE shelters was to hide special forces personnel. If the Russians attacked from the East German border, they would pass over the shelters and we would effectively be behind enemy lines and able to attack targets from behind (we ran cables into them connected to regular and night-vision cameras on nearby roads, so we could observe the movement of enemy personnel). But they were also designed to protect us from the effects of not only artillery, but also biochemical and nuclear warfare. Clearly, they would be no protection against a direct nuclear strike, but if the radioactive snow is falling, or the air is thick with chemicals or toxins, underground is often the safest place to be.

Despite being aerated by vents with charcoal filters, these MEXE shelters were horrible, cramped places to spend any serious amount of time. I knew this better than most, because I'd spent thirty-one days in one in Pontrilas, when I was an eighteen-year-old in the territorial SAS (23 SAS) and desperate for a day's wage. The Regiment wanted to know whether a six-man unit would create any kind of thermal imaging splash from above if they were in an underground shelter for this period of time. None of the lads from 22 SAS were prepared to take part in the experiment so, keen as mustard, I volunteered.

My job was to turn on and off a bank of about forty lightbulbs at various times of the day to simulate the body heat of a Regiment unit. Otherwise, I established an eight-hour on, eight-hour off stag system, lived off MREs and passed the time reading or sleeping. I was obliged to shit into plastic bags and piss into empty jerrycans. You can imagine that, after a month of that, conditions in my underground bunker were foul. And on day thirty-one, as the thermal imaging aircraft flew over the field, a farmer decided to let his sheep graze on the land, completely messing up the heat signature pattern and rendering the experiment a total waste of time. Thanks a bunch, Farmer Giles!

Biochemical and nuclear attacks affect your immediate environment, which is why underground is often your safest location. In terms of survival, much depends on your location at the time of an attack, and on the specifics of the incident. Obviously, I hope none of us ever have to make use of the information in this chapter. But these weapons exist, and there are rogue states who would be prepared to use them. There is also a risk from terrorist networks of low-level biochem attacks and improvised nuclear devices (INDs). Knowing how to act in the unlikely but ever-possible event of such an attack can mitigate the harm caused to you and your family should it occur.

BIOCHEM ATTACKS

These are attacks by biological weapons or chemical weapons. We hear of them being used by dictators in war zones, but we often assume that they are not a threat with which we need to concern ourselves. This is a mistake. Biological and chemical weapons *have* been weaponised. They *have* been used by terrorist organisations against civilian targets. It's only a matter of time before it happens again, and these weapons have the potential to cause some of the worst imaginable threats to public safety.

Dark Winter

In 2001, a number of organisations in the US simulated a terrorist biological attack to try to assess the damage it might cause. It was called Dark Winter. The Dark Winter scenario supposes that twenty people are infected by a smallpox attack in Oklahoma City. By the end of the thirteenth hypothetical day, there are 6,000 cases. After six weeks, there are 3 million infections and a million deaths.

First responders and the military get some training in responding to these kind of attacks, but the brutal reality is that a mass biochem incident has the potential to cause a disaster whose effects increase exponentially, and which the authorities will have little chance of controlling properly.

Biological weapons

These are strains of living organisms such as bacteria, viruses and fungi. It is known that organisms such as smallpox, anthrax, plague, viral equine encephalitis, botulinum and ricin have been weaponised (and this is by no means an exhaustive list). Some have vaccines, others don't. Incubation can be between a day and a month. They can cause horrific physical symptoms, and death.

Worst of all, many of these diseases can be passed from person to person. This means there is the potential for a terrorist to infect themselves on purpose and act as a 'vector', spreading the disease intentionally.

Chemical weapons

These are non-living substances intended to kill, maim or incapacitate. They are divided into:

- nerve agents – these attack the central nervous system, causing breathing difficulties, spasms and death within minutes
- blister agents – these attack and destroy the skin tissue
- blood agents – these cause convulsion, coma and cardiac arrest
- choking agents – these cause coughing, choking and respiratory problems

We would regularly train for chemical attacks in the SAS. These training sessions would involve trying to operate normally in an NBC – nuclear, biological and chemical warfare – kit. These comprised full body suits, tight plastic gloves, rubber boots to go over our regular boots, and respirators. It was the respirators that the guys hated the most. On one training exercise, a few of them removed the filters from their mask so they could breathe more easily on a ten-mile march. They regretted doing this when our instructors hit us with a CR gas attack. The guys with undamaged respirators were fine. The guys who had doctored theirs were on their knees and coughing their guts up.

These suits and respirators are your best defence against chemical weapons attacks, but they're not really appropriate to a civilian situation.

How are they dispersed?

Biological and chemical weapons can be dispersed using 'line source' systems – this would most likely be from a light aircraft – or 'point source' systems, which would most likely be small exploding packages. The latter is more likely. This was the dispersal system of the 1995 sarin attack on the Tokyo underground, which killed thirteen people but injured thousands of others. We can't discount line-source dispersal systems, however. An al-Qaeda operative is known to have questioned Florida crop dusters about the spray systems on their aircraft. No prizes for guessing what he had in mind.

As always, the first line of defence against a biochem attack – especially a 'point source' attack – is situational awareness. When train announcers tell you to beware of suspicious packages, don't only think in terms of bombs and IEDs. Think biochem dispersal units.

Indicators of a biochem attack

You may not be instantly aware that a biochem attack has occurred. There are certain indicators:

- Unexplained smells, especially the smell of newly mown grass or bitter almonds.
- Dead animals, fish, birds and insects.
- Dead grass, trees or plants when there is no drought.
- Unexplained metallic debris, especially if it seems to have contained a liquid, or looks like abandoned spraying devices.
- Physical symptoms in yourself or others, such as blistered skin, swellings, choking and respiratory difficulties.
- Unexplained drops of liquid on surfaces when there has been no rain.
- Unexplained oily film on water surfaces.

What to do in the event of a biochem attack

Your first line of defence is non-exposure. If a biochem attack is announced by the emergency services or the media, get indoors. As far as possible, isolate yourself from other people. Tape up the gaps around your door frames and windows. Seal your fireplace. You are aiming to make your house a sealed unit.

Fill your bath, sinks and as many vessels as you can with water. Biochem attacks can affect the water supply, so you want to get your stocks up before that happens.

In extreme cases, you may need to hole up for long periods of time, in which case the information below on sheltering from nuclear fallout applies.

Monitor the media carefully. There will be advice on symptoms to look out for depending on the substance used in the attack, and instructions on what to do if you exhibit these symptoms.

If you are on the street or in a public area in the event of a biochem attack, you need to simulate the protection of an NBC suit. Tuck your trousers into your socks. Try to cover all parts of your skin. Breathe through an old T-shirt or a piece of cloth to mimic a respirator's filter. Evacuate the area, trying to move at right angles to the direction of the wind, so you are moving away from the direction of gas or toxins.

If you believe you've had contact with these weapons, get to a hospital immediately. Your life may depend on how quickly you receive medical treatment.

NUCLEAR ATTACKS

When people imagine a nuclear attack, they generally suppose that major cities such as London or New York are the most likely initial targets. This may be the case, but there are other likely targets such as RAF bases, naval and submarine bases, communications centres and broadcasting centres. In the event of a nuclear-strike advance warning, avoid these locations.

In order to understand our best responses to a nuclear strike, we must first understand what happens when a nuclear device detonates. The effect of a nuclear explosion can be divided into three categories: the blast damage, the electromagnetic pulse and the fallout.

Blast damage

If you're at, or near, ground zero of a nuclear strike, you're dead. The intensity of the explosion and the high temperature of the resulting fireball will incinerate buildings and humans. The further away you are from ground zero, the higher your chances of survival from thermal injuries. I can't tell you how far away you need to be to survive, because there are too many factors involved such as the size of the bomb, the position above the level of the earth that the bomb detonates, and the number of tall buildings between you and the thermal blast. The maps below will give you an idea of the distances involved.

It is worth knowing, however, that there are two components to the blast: the thermal pulse and the blast wave. The thermal pulse is a blinding flash of light. The blast wave is the outward burst of air from the explosion. The thermal pulse travels faster than the blast wave. If you're at a substantial distance from ground zero – we're talking several miles – this means you'll see the pulse a few seconds before the blast wave hits. Those few seconds may give you enough time to seek cover and protect yourself from the effects of the blast, such as flying debris and glass.

EMP

The EMP is an electromagnetic pulse that occurs with detonation of a nuclear device. It poses no threat to humans, but it does damage electronic equipment – including some vehicles, fuel pumps, street and domestic lighting and comms equipment. This will affect your ability to communicate with the outside world if you are sheltering from nuclear fallout, and to escape if you make the decision to run (see below).

Radiation

There are two types of radiation after a nuclear explosion: initial radiation and residual radiation.

Initial radiation is that which arrives within a minute of the blast. Its strength decreases quickly with distance from ground zero. Most people who receive lethal doses of initial radiation will be killed by the blast anyway.

Residual radiation comes from the nuclear fallout – radioactive particles that fall to earth over a wide area surrounding the blast. It consists mostly of beta and gamma radiation, and can be hazardous for months or years afterward. Sometimes the fallout cannot be seen, but it normally settles between one and twenty-four hours of the blast.

Your chances of surviving the blast damage of a nuclear explosion are directly related to how far you are from ground zero, and how big the bomb is. To give you an idea of the distances involved, I'm going to tell you the approximate effects of two different types of bomb. One is a 100-kiloton bomb (this is the size of the W-76 bomb, common in the UK's nuclear arsenal), one is a 100-megaton bomb (this is the size of the 'Tsar Bomba', currently the largest Russian nuke). I'm assuming the bomb explodes on the ground rather than in the air. (Note that these figures can only ever be approximate.)

	100 kiloton bomb	*100 megaton bomb*
Fireball radius	500 metres	4.9 miles
Radiation radius (causing up to 90% mortality between several hours and several weeks)	1.1 miles	4.3 miles
Air blast radius (causing buildings to collapse and extensive fatalities)	1.3 miles	13.2 miles
Thermal radiation radius (causing third-degree burns)	2.4 miles	39.9 miles
Distance fallout can travel with a 15 mph wind	115 miles	1019 miles

To give you an idea of what these distances mean, here are the relative effects shown on maps of London, Birmingham and Glasgow (the fallout distances aren't shown, because they are dependent on the prevailing winds). You need to get out of the outer circle to have a chance of surviving the blast.

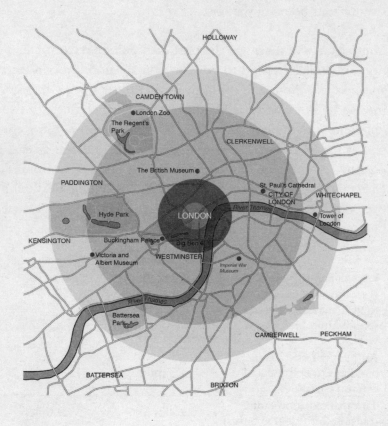

HOLLOWAY

CAMDEN TOWN

London Zoo

The Regent's
Park

CLERKENWELL

The British Museum

PADDINGTON

St. Paul's Cathedral
CITY OF
LONDON

WHITECHAPEL

River Thames

LONDON

Tower of
London

Hyde Park

KENSINGTON

Buckingham Palace

Big Ben

Victoria and
Albert Museum

WESTMINSTER

Imperial War
Museum

River Thames

Battersea
Park

CAMBERWELL

PECKHAM

BATTERSEA

BRIXTON

Radiation radius

Fireball radius

Air blast radius

Thermal radiation radius

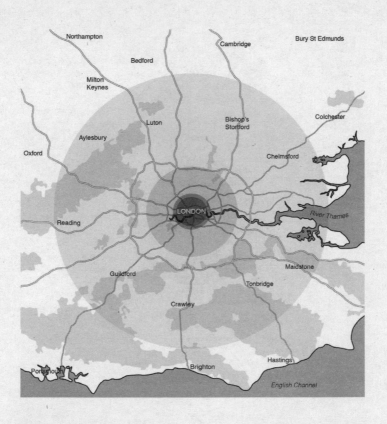

Radiation radius

Fireball radius

Air blast radius

Thermal radiation radius

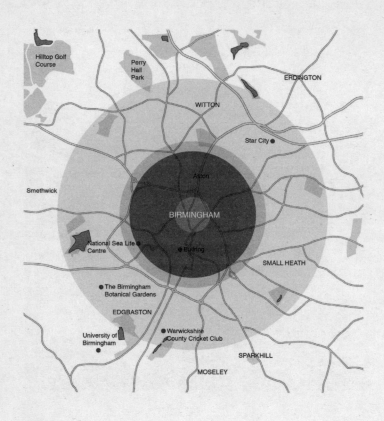

Hilltop Golf
Course

Perry
Hall
Park

ERDINGTON

WITTON

Star City ●

Aston

Smethwick

BIRMINGHAM

National Sea Life
Centre ●

● Bullring

SMALL HEATH

● The Birmingham
Botanical Gardens

EDGBASTON

University of
Birmingham
●

● Warwickshire
County Cricket Club

SPARKHILL

MOSELEY

● Radiation radius

● Fireball radius

● Air blast radius

● Thermal radiation radius

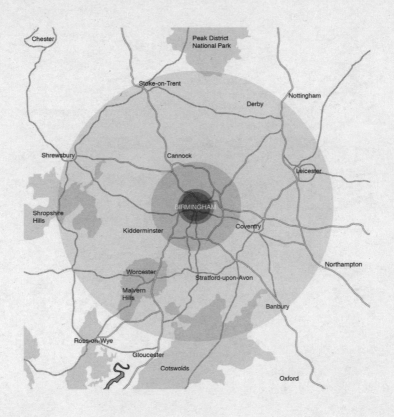

- Radiation radius
- Fireball radius
- Air blast radius
- Thermal radiation radius

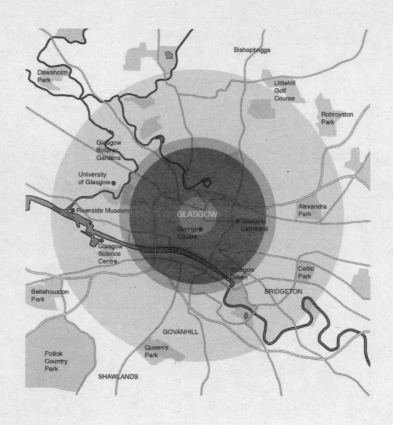

Radiation radius

Fireball radius

Air blast radius

Thermal radiation radius

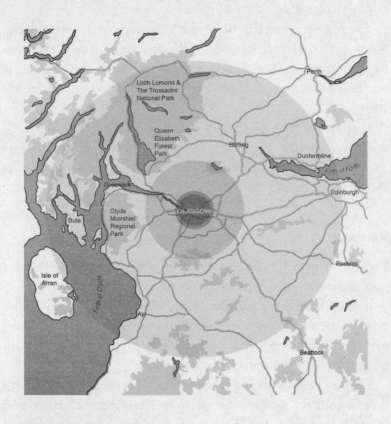

- Radiation radius
- Fireball radius
- Air blast radius
- Thermal radiation radius

For comparison, the Hiroshima bomb was fifteen kilotons – much smaller than either of these.

You can see from this how much depends on the size of the bomb. You need to be outside of the thermal radiation radius to have a realistic chance of survival, so in the event of a 100-megaton bomb warning, you must get at *least* sixty-five kilometres away.

However, if you do survive, you have a choice to make: do you try to outrun the nuclear fallout, or do you shelter from it?

Here are the elements I would consider when running or sheltering from a nuclear attack.

Running

Perhaps there has been a warning of a nuclear attack. Perhaps you've survived the blast but want to escape the fallout.

If there has been a warning, be prepared for mass panic. The chances are that in such a scenario, the authorities will make all exit routes from high-risk areas one way only, but you must still be prepared for crowds, chaos and looting.

Keep away from major cities, military installations and towns with a military connection such as Hereford, Aldershot and High Wycombe. I would advise you to head for unpopulated areas: deserted countryside and moors. These are the areas least likely to be targeted.

If you have survived a blast and have decided to run to escape the fallout, you need to be aware that vehicles and public transport may have been put out of action by the EMP. This means you'll be on foot. The chances of putting much distance between yourself and the fallout aren't great. If you *do* run, try to identify the direction of the wind. Use this, and your knowledge of the position of ground zero, to calculate the best direction to run. But in this event your safest course of action will probably be to find shelter. Do it quickly: if you've survived this far, your best chance of continued survival is to get shelter from the fallout within sixty minutes.

Sheltering

If you've had warning of a nuclear attack and you're outside of the expected blast radius, you may well decide not to run and to prioritise sheltering from the fallout. You will have only a short window of time. Your priorities will be: a substantial physical barrier between you and any radioactive fallout; water; personal hygiene; food; communications. These priorities hold if you are sheltering quickly having survived an unexpected blast, but clearly, you'll have less time to make the necessary arrangements.

Substantial physical barrier

Radiation can penetrate solid barriers, but the thicker the barrier, the more resistant it is to radiation. You need to put as much solid material between yourself and the fallout as possible. This is where underground shelters come in, and it is why underground nuclear bunkers are encased in thick walls of concrete.

If your house has a cellar, get down there. Otherwise, get to the structurally strongest part of the building – this is often under the stairs. Tape up all doors and windows. If possible, surround yourself with mattresses, filing cabinets, bookcases.

Barricade yourself and your family in to get the best protection possible from the fallout.

Water

You might be in this shelter for weeks before the emergency services get to you (though be aware that the radioactive effects of the fallout on the outside world can last for months or years). The amount of time you can survive will depend on the quantity of water you have. Fill every vessel in your house with water. Do it quickly, before the water supplies become contaminated. Stockpile bottled water if you have the opportunity to get your hands on it. Ration this water carefully – it is your lifeline.

Personal hygiene

An SAS man learns a lot about personal hygiene in the jungle. You won't last two weeks there if you don't look after your body. It starts falling to pieces. The same will happen in a sealed-off cellar, or whatever you are using as a nuclear shelter.

When I was in that MEXE shelter for thirty-one days as an eighteen-year-old, I was obliged to urinate into a jerrycan and defecate into plastic bags, which I would then double wrap and seal. This is what you will need to do in a nuclear shelter. I was meticulous about my hygiene, but after I had emerged, I washed my body thoroughly and then returned to the clothes I'd been wearing. The smell of shit was overpowering: a reminder that the microbes of human waste hang in the air and cling to everything. You must be scrupulous about personal hygiene if you are to avoid debilitating sickness.

Try to get some wet wipes into your shelter. Use these to clean your body regularly, especially under your arms and your